Military
Fitness

Military Fitness

PATRICK DALE

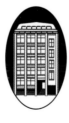

ROBERT HALE • LONDON

ISBN 978-0-7090-9314-5

Robert Hale Limited
Clerkenwell House
Clerkenwell Green
London EC1R 0HT

www.halebooks.com

A catalogue record for this book is available from the British Library

2 4 6 8 10 9 7 5 3 1

Printed in China

Contents

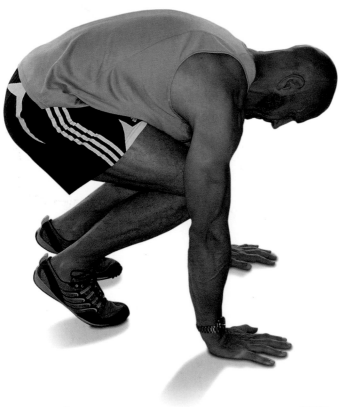

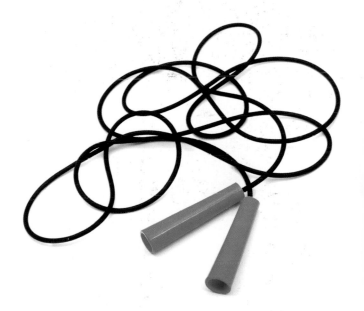

Introduction
Military fitness, past and present

Military Fitness through the Ages

Throughout history, men and women have fought to extend their territories, to protect their homelands from hostile invaders, to preserve their culture and way of life and to defend weaker neighbours from oppression. For every outstanding fighting force, from the Spartans and the Roman legions to the modern-day Navy SEALs and the Royal Marine Commandos, fitness has played a vital role in the success of many military operations.

Modern soldiers need a wide number of fitness attributes.

History is littered with amazing stories of exceptional military fitness: the Spartans of Greece and the legions of Rome marched hundreds – sometimes thousands

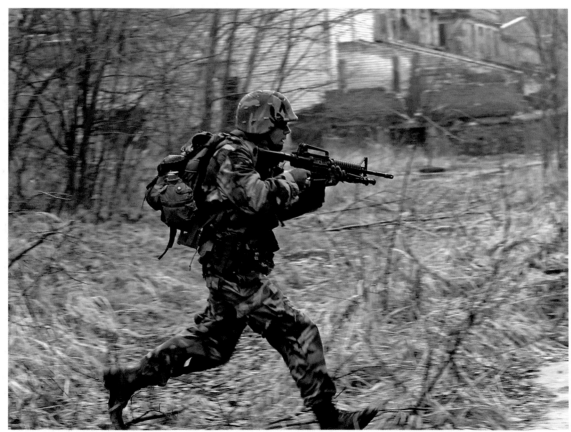

- of miles to reach their respective enemies and then fought in brutal hand-to-hand combat where strength, power and endurance would often be the difference between life and a bloody death. The ability of the Romans to march almost incomprehensible distances while fighting regular battles saw the Roman Empire expand massively. The Spartans, a race of Greek warriors, trained their bodies from an early age to be supremely capable on the battlefield. At the Battle of Thermopylae in 480BC, 300 Spartan warriors held off tens of thousands of Persians for seven days before finally being defeated in what has been described by military experts as one of the most epic last stands in history. During his reign of virtual dominance of the ancient world, Alexander the Great's armies marched tens of thousands of miles across some of the most inhospitable terrain to be found in that era.

Knights of the Middle Ages were also renowned for their physical prowess. Fighting in heavy armour and wielding long swords, maces, battleaxes and shields took tremendous muscular endurance, core strength, balance, fitness and power, and feats of knightly valour are all the more impressive when it is remembered that armour could weigh in excess of 25 kg. Knights trained from a very early age to

Medieval combat was a true test of muscle and might!

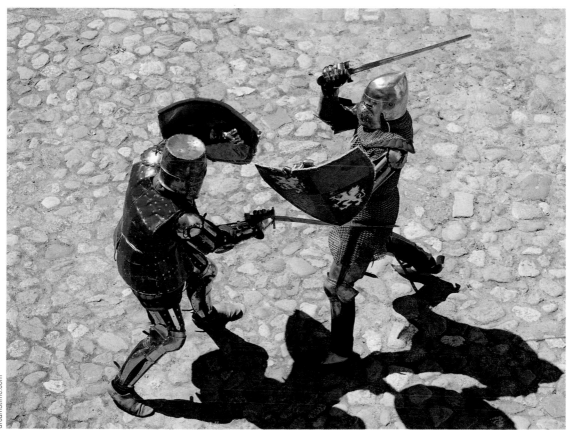

dreamstime.com

develop the necessary conditioning to survive the rigours of medieval combat and when not at war – a rarity at the time – most knights kept their fitness and skills honed by competing in military contests against other knights, including jousting and duelling for honour, sport and money.

More recent feats of militaristic fitness and might include the epic 'Falklands march' undertaken by Royal Marine Commandos who, on 21 May 1982, marched 90 km (56 miles) carrying in excess of 36 kg (80 lb) of kit per man over some of the most arduous terrain in order to engage a superior number of Argentinian soldiers. Not only did the Marines win the battle – a major turning point in the Falklands conflict – but, on completion of the fight and without respite, they 'lifted and shifted' straight on to higher ground to secure the area and defend the position from further attack. This type of heavily laden forced march is called yomping in Marine-speak and is one of the unique workouts included in the military fitness solutions 12-week programme in Chapter 5.

Although the weapons and theatres of war have changed dramatically since the days of Sparta and Rome, the demands placed on the modern soldier's body are virtually identical. The Russian Spetsnaz, American Delta Force, French Foreign Legion, British Parachute Regiment, Royal Marine Commandos and other elite military forces around the world all share the common bond of supreme physical fitness with their ancient counterparts. Despite technological advancements in both transport and weaponry, modern soldiers need to be just as supremely fit as the Roman foot soldiers, Spartan warriors and knights of long ago.

The Military Total Fitness Model

Military fitness means being fit for anything. As a member of an elite military team you could be hacking through dense jungle one day, cross-country skiing the next and battling through the urban sprawl of a city ruined by heavy shelling the day after that. Being militarily fit means you have to be versatile. Strength without fitness, or fitness without agility and quickness, is of little use and your all-round fitness may be all that ensures your survival.

Lots of us want to 'get fit', but fitness means different things to different people. This leads to a lot of wasted workouts and poor progress as exercisers strive to achieve something they have not clearly defined. In actuality, fitness is the successful adaptation to physical stress. Physical fitness is specific – you get fitter according to the training you perform on a regular basis. If you lift weights, you get stronger. If you run a long way, you improve your cardiovascular conditioning. If you stretch frequently, you'll increase your flexibility. If, however, you want to improve your fitness so that you can cope with a wider variety of demands than just lifting weights, long-distance running or performing feats of contortion, you need to train in a variety of ways. This is called cross-training and encapsulates the very spirit of military fitness.

The components of a military total fitness model include:

- Strength
- Power
- Endurance
- Aerobic fitness
- Anaerobic fitness
- Flexibility
- Core strength
- Balance, coordination and agility – collectively called athleticism

The workouts in this book will improve every aspect of your fitness and will equip you with all of the physical attributes you need to be militarily fit – in other words, they will enable you to develop fitness with purpose.

Bodybuilders – not always as strong as they look!

What it Means to be Militarily Fit

Being militarily fit means being fit for anything life throws at you. Military fitness will allow you to hike or run long distances while carrying equipment if necessary. You'll be strong enough to perform chin-ups, dips, sit-ups, lunges and squats with ease as well as a host of other bodyweight and strength-training exercises. You will be agile and athletic and able to sprint, jump, climb and crawl over obstacles and your ability to keep going despite being fatigued will make you the envy of just about anyone who ever wants to join you for a workout. While some exercisers prefer to specialize, and emphasize only one or two of the components that make up a well-rounded model of fitness, military fitness is all-encompassing and truly functional. Consider these three typical approaches to exercise: bodybuilding, long-distance running and yoga – each popular and effective in its own right but also highly restrictive in terms of functional cross-training benefits.

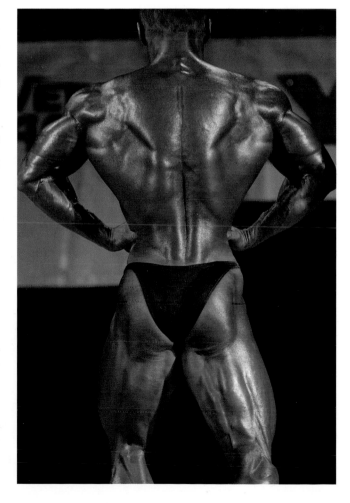

Bodybuilding develops strength and muscle size but places no emphasis on aerobic or anaerobic conditioning, mobility, flexibility, athleticism or agility. Bodybuilding training often targets muscles in isolation as opposed to working the body as a whole synergistic unit – which is how it actually works. A bodybuilder may be strong and look fit, but the reality is often that it's 'all show and no go'! Don't worry though – despite this anti-bodybuilding rhetoric, if you follow the exercises detailed in this book, you'll still develop muscle in all the right places. Furthermore, you'll not just *look* strong, you'll *be* strong too!

Long-distance runners are aerobically fit but the reality is that, while they have the heart and lungs of a thoroughbred racehorse, they often lack strength, speed, power, agility and flexibility. A long-distance runner might win the race to the finishing line but, once the running is done and the fighting starts, will often lack the strength to put the enemy down. To be a successful long-distance runner you need to be light and slightly muscled, which is ideal for covering long distances quickly but a real drawback if you have to carry 25 kg of essential kit on your back, or go toe-to-toe with the enemy. The programme in this book will develop a supreme level of aerobic fitness but, unlike the archetypal distance runner, you'll also be able to sprint, jump, climb and lift should the need arise.

Yoga develops flexibility in the extreme.

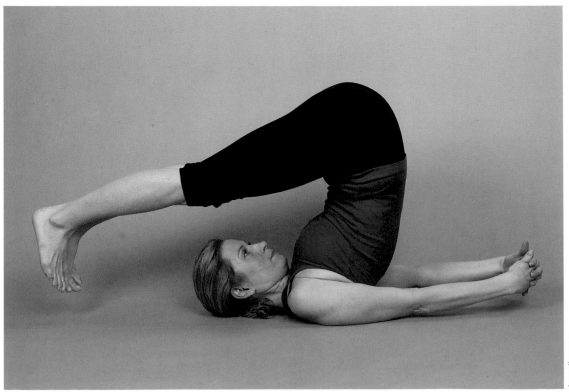

dreamstime.com

Military Fitness

Yoga develops tremendous flexibility and can be very healthful but, as a rule, when you sprint, climb, jump, crawl or lift heavy objects you use your muscles quickly and not in the controlled, slow, rhythmic way that typifies yoga. It's all well and good being able to contort your body while you are in a relaxed state and your breathing is under control but the reality is that military life is more demanding and unpredictable. Also, yoga does not develop aerobic fitness, high degrees of strength, power or athleticism. During this programme we'll be working on your flexibility – it's essential for the health of your joints and muscles, as well as for helping you avoid injury – but you'll be focusing on *dynamic flexibility* or, in other words, flexibility when you are on the move.

As you can see, while each of these common training methods offers selective benefits, on its own none of them will provide the all-round type of fitness that means you'll be fit for whatever life throws at you. Each one leaves something out of the military total fitness model. That type of fitness can only be developed by using a holistic approach to training that treats your body as a single, complex synergistic unit rather than a collection of parts and systems to be broken down and worked in isolation.

To summarize, being militarily fit will allow you to perform a wide range of physical activities well. You might not be as strong as a bodybuilder, as running-fit as a distance runner, or as flexible as a yoga practitioner but you'll be able to hold your own in almost any physically demanding situation where multiple fitness attributes are required at the same time. Your high level of fitness will make you a great all-rounder, ready for anything and, most importantly, you'll have no weaknesses in your fitness component arsenal.

The Military Fitness Look

While looking good might not be the aim of military fitness training, the men and women of the elite armed forces have some of the best physiques around. They look as though they are ready for anything and their bodies function as well as they look. A militarily fit body is stripped down, lithe and athletic – strong but not bulky and without the comic-book muscles of the bodybuilder. Lean, but not skinny like a long-distance runner, the physiques of elite soldiers are the result of a combination of training approaches that borrow from just about every form of exercise and extract only the best and most useful methods from each. A hybrid approach to fitness, military training selects training methods based on results. If it doesn't work it is quickly discarded.

By following the advice and exercise programmes in this book you can be assured that your fabulously well-functioning body will also look amazing – you'll start to look like an athlete, although observers may find it hard to decide which sport you compete in. Opinions will range from boxer to decathlete but the consensus will be that you look 'fit for anything'! Expect to turn heads at the beach – and not because it looks as though you have swallowed a beach ball!

Getting Lean, Looking Mean

The training outlined in this book will get you lean, make you real-world strong, increase your all-round fitness and transform your body from civilian-soft to military-hard. You'll get leaner than you ever dreamed of and reveal muscles you didn't know you had. Although none of the workouts have been designed specifically as fat-burners (you'll find very little mention of the fat-burning zone in this book) you'll be incinerating plenty of calories during each of the specially designed training sessions which, combined with the dietary advice in Chapter 7, will get you lean and keep you lean without the need for long, boring workouts or overly restrictive and unpleasant eating plans. You'll be making use of our secret weapon called EPOC in the battle against body fat, but you'll learn more about this in later chapters.

Unlike the emaciated runner or bulked-up bodybuilder, you'll look as good in regular clothes as you do in your bathing suit or workout gear. A narrow waist, broad shoulders, excellent posture and increased all-round confidence will give you an aura of fitness and health that positively radiates physical prowess and vitality.

If weight loss is your primary goal, you'll find the workouts in the 12-week programme brutally effective for stripping away body fat. Combining this with the in-depth nutritional advice included in Chapter 7, you'll be on your way to looking lean, mean and athletic.

Getting with the Programme

The military fitness programme grows with you. Session by session, week by week, as your fitness levels increase the workouts will press you just a little bit harder. Like the tough but fair drill sergeant or physical training instructor, the programme will ask you to work a little harder each week to improve your fitness levels beyond anything you previously imagined was possible. Each workout has been designed to develop real-world fitness, endurance and strength. The programmes don't include any pumping, toning or isolation exercises for minor muscle groups, or complicated training systems that leave your brain sorer than your muscles. Instead you'll be performing plenty of tried and tested exercises and workouts that have successfully served military men and women for many years and have stood the test of time. Don't let the simplicity of the exercises or programmes fool you though – what military fitness training lacks in complexity is more than made up for by intensity and intent.

All of the workouts are scalable so you can tailor them to fit your individual fitness level. You'll get plenty of advice on how to change the workouts to meet your current needs and abilities. Many of the workouts are 'against the clock' so you'll be working at your own pace with a view to bettering your performance over subsequent workouts. Unless you reach your genetic potential – and very few people ever do – you'll find that your fitness increases each week, month and year you follow this programme. Once you have experienced the benefits of this kind of uncomplicated, effective training, you'll never go back to traditional low-intensity, spot-targeting, resistance machine-based, ineffective workouts again.

Your Standing Orders

Each workout is preceded by a thorough and effective warm-up which will help to prepare your body for the coming session and make sure you can perform at your best. Likewise, you'll finish each workout with a cool-down to return your body to its pre-exercise state. Think of the warm-up and cool-down as being standing orders – they are not optional! Failure to follow a standing order can result in court martial and failure to warm up and cool down may result in injury. Smart soldiers avoid both! Details on how to warm up and cool down properly, as well as a whole host of other flexibility and stretching information, can be found in Chapter 4.

Simply Effective, Effectively Simple

The exercises contained within the workouts are military standards that are used all over the globe to develop phenomenal levels of fitness. Many of the exercises have been around for centuries, unlike so many of the fads you'll see performed in gyms today. Although there are more high-tech approaches that you can use to get fit, the simple Spartanesque, streamlined approach to fitness is one of the best ways to get naturally fit and strong. There is nothing wrong with technological advancement but over-reliance on technology can cause you serious problems in battle and in exercise ... you never know when you might find yourself behind enemy lines with nothing but your wits and the things you find around you for equipment.

In terms of exercise, by limiting the use of complicated and expensive exercise equipment you will learn the art of 'survival fitness'. That is to say, you'll develop the ability to use your surrounding area as the workout area and your body as a gym.

The simplicity of the workouts in this programme means that you'll never need to miss a workout because of a queue for the treadmill or because someone else is using the leg extension machine. You'll be able to perform your workouts virtually anywhere and anytime. As a Royal Marine, I spent lots of time training in some very unusual locations and despite less than optimal surroundings still maintained very high levels of combat fitness. Even now, as a gym owner, I seldom use more than a few free weights, a skipping rope and some floor space to maintain a similar level of fitness to when I was on deployment.

You may, in fact, find that you are better served by spending the money you would normally spend on your gym subscription on buying a few pieces of workout kit to use in the privacy of your own home. You will also find details in Chapter 6 on how to make your own workout gear for next to nothing if you prefer not to spend much money on workout equipment.

So, without further ado, turn the page and take your first step towards developing military fitness that will make you fit for whatever life (and the enemy) throws at you!

CHAPTER ONE

Your Military Fitness Exercise Brief
Establishing the principles

When it comes to getting in great shape, it seems as though everyone is an expert. Just trawl the internet and you'll see what I mean. The thing is, most of these so-called experts are usually trying to sell you a fancy or complicated piece of exercise equipment or a brand new state-of-the-art supplement, or to get you to subscribe to their website for further information! The reality is that getting in great shape – fit enough for just about anything – requires very little in the way of equipment and, while supplements may help, they are by no means the essential purchase you may have been led to believe. To get fitter than you ever imagined possible, all that you need to do is follow some simple exercise principles. You *will* have to work hard but then nothing worth having ever came easy – just ask any Royal Marine Commando about basic training to confirm that!

The tools of the trade for developing strength

The Exercise Principles

So, what is fitness? Fitness is the successful physical adaptation to stress, and this concept is commonly abbreviated to SAID, which stands for Specific Adaptations to Imposed Demands. Exercise challenges the systems of your body and your body responds by getting fitter and stronger. The thing is, though, if you only ever lift the same weights, run the same distances or perform the identical number of repetitions (reps), you'll never get any fitter. If you want your fitness levels to sky-rocket to stratospheric heights, you'll need to 'screw the nut' from time to time and make sure you push yourself a little harder from one workout to the next. For exercise to result in successful adaptations, you need to observe the training principles that follow. Observing these principles will mean that you will be continually challenging your body and, consequently, you *will* get fitter.

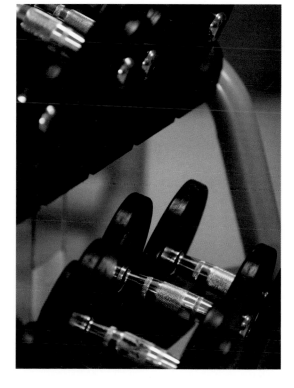

1. **Overload** - this means doing more than you are used to and ties in with the SAID principle discussed above. You need to do a little more than the previous time so that your workouts provide a greater challenge to the systems of your body. We'll look at how you go about doing this a little later when we discuss the training variables.

2. **Adaptation** - adaptations are specific to the type of exercise you perform. If you lift heavy weights you will get stronger and if you run long distances you will get fitter. It's important to realize at this point that military fitness is not a small spectrum of fitness characteristics but, in fact, covers the entire A to Z of fitness. While strength is admirable, it's of little use on the battlefield if you have to rest every 30 seconds because of poor cardiovascular fitness! The programme contained in this book is specifically designed to improve *all* of the fitness components so that you are 'jack of all trades'. This may mean that you will have a few favourite workouts and others that you are less enthused about but, as a hard-but-fair Physical Training Instructor would say: 'Suck it up, Lofty'!

3. **Reversibility** - simply put, fitness is a 'use it or lose it' commodity - you can't *store* fitness. This means that breaks from your training programme will probably result in a loss of fitness and strength. A day off here and there will not do you any harm (it may, in fact, be beneficial) but long breaks in training will result in regression rather than progression - the opposite of what we are trying to achieve. If possible, stick with the programme in this book as closely as you can and avoid taking prolonged breaks from training. If you do have to break up the programme, I strongly suggest that you go back a few weeks so that you can regain some of your lost fitness. You *could* jump back in at the point where you stopped but this may result in injury and will definitely result in fatigue and muscle soreness.

4. **Recovery** - at the risk of sounding like a contradiction, the principle of recovery means that you must take periodic breaks from training. Your body goes through its adaptive process during periods of rest. Your workouts break you down so you have to allow time for your body to build back up and repair itself. This happens at night while you sleep, and on your days off from training. Your body also gets the opportunity for rest and recovery when you train in different ways on different days. By mixing up your workouts throughout the week you avoid overloading any one specific system. With that in mind, keep the workouts in the order they have been laid out in the programme - if you alter the order you may find that you put two similar workouts back-to-back and hinder your progress.

5. **Overtraining** – in the golden age of bodybuilding, some experts suggested that there was no such thing as overtraining but merely under-eating. While this may have been true for the guys living on muscle beach, whose lives revolved around training, eating, sleeping and sunbathing, for the rest of us who have to balance our personal and professional lives with our fitness aspirations, overtraining is a real risk. If you start to lose enthusiasm for your workouts, lack energy, find that your sleep is disrupted in any way, lose your appetite, ache constantly or seem to be suffering more colds or illnesses than usual, you may be overtraining. If you experience any of these symptoms, immediately reduce the volume and intensity of your workouts for a few days, increase your intake of healthy vitamin- and mineral-packed foods and examine other aspects of your life for crossover stresses. If your work or home life is especially challenging or you find yourself pulled in lots of directions at once, consider reducing your training intensity and volume until you feel better able to cope with the demands of your workouts. Many promising sporting careers have been derailed by overtraining, so, if in doubt, take your foot off the gas for a while. Overtraining is better avoided than treated. Overtraining is discussed in depth in Chapter 8.

6. **Progression** – this is the key to continued fitness developments. The programme in this book is progressive and will push you to develop greater levels of fitness and strength over the coming weeks and months. As you find yourself getting into better and better shape, you will also need to take responsibility for your fitness progress by adapting the prescribed workouts. Remember points 1 and 2 above – you have to ask more of your body if you want it to respond with increased levels of fitness and strength. Progression should be linear and logical and relies on your manipulation of the training variables which are discussed below.

The Exercise Variables

Strategic and logical manipulation of the training variables is the key to your long-term fitness success. It would be very easy to design a workout that, in military terms, 'thrashes you to within an inch of your life', but one-off 'beastings' do very little to improve your fitness. It's more a case of making small changes over a prolonged time rather than doubling your workload overnight. One of the most important skills of a Physical Trainer is to be able to push your recruits (and you are my recruit) as hard as possible without actually pushing them over the edge and into demoralizing failure. This means making small, subtle but regular changes to your workouts.

I'm often asked whether exercise ever gets any easier and my answer is a resounding 'No'! All that happens is your work capacity increases in line with your fitness. A beginner and an advanced exerciser can be working equally hard – it's just that the advanced exerciser is capable of producing more measurable work as he or she runs faster or lifts heavier weights. I've been exercising for over 25 years but, like any raw recruit, I still get DOMS (Delayed Onset Muscle Soreness) when I overextend myself or try something new – it's part and parcel of striving for increased fitness and strength.

The following are your exercising variables. Think of them as things that you can alter within your workouts to keep your levels of strength and fitness progressing.

1. **Increased number of exercises per muscle group** - instead of performing just press-ups for your chest, add dips into the mix as well. This will add to the overall volume of your workout and result in increased fitness gains.

2. **Increased number of sets** - another way to add more volume to your workouts is to perform more sets of each exercise. While extra volume is an effective way of increasing the challenge of your workouts, there is a finite amount of training volume that your body can cope with. Always ask yourself: 'Is more volume necessary or am I better off increasing intensity?'

3. **Increased repetitions** - some exercises such as press-ups and pull-ups use a fixed resistance, so you should strive to get your numbers up as you get fitter. As with the previous point, there comes a time when more repetitions are not very effective so you may need to look at ways to make your training sessions harder rather than longer.

4. **Increased exercise intensity** - you can make exercises harder in a number of ways. With strength training you can simply add more weight to the bar and with cardiovascular (cardio) work you can increase your pace, but there are plenty of other ways in which you can intensify your workouts. As a general rule, performing more than 20 repetitions of a given exercise is not an effective use of your time and you will actually get fitter faster by training harder as opposed to longer.

5. **Increased frequency of exercise** - training more often can help you get fitter, but only up to a point. Training *too* frequently can result in overtraining. If you are a beginner, you may find that three to four workouts a week is ideal initially, but you may work up to five or six workouts a week as you get fitter. Always bear in mind that rest days are just as important as training days and they are when your body builds up and recovers from the rigours of your workouts. The key to successful exercise is training enough to elicit the fitness response you desire, but not so often that workouts lose their effectiveness.

6. **Exercise variety** – a change is as good as a rest, or so they say. Your body is a master adapter and will look for ways to make the exercises you perform easier. By now you know that easier exercises do not a fitter recruit make! To avoid this, use a variety of exercises to work your body in lots of different ways. Mixing exercise modalities will keep your body 'guessing' and therefore adapting. However, don't become a workout butterfly and change your programme so often that your body doesn't get a chance to adapt at all. Some consistency is necessary.

7. **Exercise complexity** – sometimes, trickier exercises are one of the best ways to make progress. For example, if you are stuck on sets of 20 press-ups and don't seem to be able to make any progress, switch to balance ball press-ups for a few weeks, When you return to regular press-ups you will find them much easier to perform than before.

8. **Exercise stability** – the less stable your base of support, the more challenging an exercise becomes. You can increase the balance demand of your exercises by performing single-limbed exercises (for example one-legged squats), reducing your base of support (for example performing shoulder presses standing on one leg), or using balance balls. Increasing the stability demands of an exercise results in tougher exercises without necessarily increasing the load you are using.

9. **Decreased rest between sets** – rest is a necessary part of any workout and allows you to regain your strength ready for the next set. Systematically knocking off a few seconds of rest here and there places a much greater demand on your recovery abilities and can make any workout much more demanding. This training variable works well with strength training and cardio intervals and results in an increased density of work, i.e. more work performed in less time.

10. **Greater exercise duration** – this variable specifically refers to cardio exercises. According to the principle of specificity, if you want to be able to exercise for longer, you have to exercise for longer! However, there is a point of diminishing returns at which *too great* an exercise duration becomes counterproductive. To give you an example, Royal Marines' basic training culminates in a 48 km (30 mile) forced march across the rough terrain of Dartmoor. The recruits seldom perform training that gets even close to this distance and yet more recruits pass this test than fail. Obviously, this is in part down to the recruits' 'never say die' attitude, but there is also the fact that, although they might never have covered such a distance before, the intensity and frequency of their workouts in the preceding weeks has equipped them to be able to cope with this sort of challenge. The bottom line is – don't go overboard with exercise duration, as intensity is actually the more useful training variable.

Exercise Terminology

Like the military, exercise experts use a lot of specialist terminology so, to help you navigate the programmes that come later, here is a glossary of common exercise terms. While there won't be a vocabulary test at the end of this chapter, you'll see many of these terms over and over throughout the book, so it will pay to commit them to memory.

1. **Repetition (commonly shortened to rep)** - a complete movement of a given exercise.

2. **Set** - a group of repetitions.

3. **Repetition maximum (RM)** - if the maximum weight you can lift twice is 20kg, 20kg is your 2RM. A weight you can lift once but not twice would be defined as your 1RM and is a measure of true strength.

4. **Intensity** - has a number of definitions that are fairly interchangeable. Intensity can be used to describe how hard an exercise feels, the load in relationship to your 1RM or how hard you have to drive yourself to complete a workout, i.e. mental intensity.

5. **Volume** - the number of sets performed during a workout. Some of your workouts will be very short, intense and low volume, whereas others may involve moderate or higher volume.

6. **Tempo** - the speed at which exercises should be performed. This may vary from a 6-second lift followed by a 6-second lower, to explosive exercises that take barely a second to perform. When in doubt, perform your exercises more slowly rather than faster. Slow-tempo exercise is much more demanding as your muscles are under tension for longer. Obviously, aerobic exercise is the exception to this principle - see Chapter 3 for more on this subject.

7. **Compound exercise** - exercises that involve movement around a number of joints simultaneously are called compound exercises. Compound exercises tend to have more real-world carryover and develop usable strength. Press-ups, squats, lunges, dead lifts and pull-ups are all examples of compound exercises.

8. **Isolation exercise** - exercises where movement is restricted to single joints are called isolation exercises. Isolation exercises target one or very few muscles at a time and are common in bodybuilding programmes. You'll be performing very few isolation exercises as they do not provide much 'bang for your buck'.

9. **Hypertrophy/Anabolism** – hypertrophy describes the enlargement of tissues which occurs through the process of anabolism – think anabolic steroids. You'll experience hypertrophy in your major muscles but, unlike the bodybuilder, your muscles will get stronger as well as bigger. Big muscles are all well and good but, if they're all show and no go, you'll soon be left behind during military manoeuvres.

10. **Atrophy/Catabolism** – atrophy is the breaking down of tissue that can occur as a result of inactivity, incapacitation or injury. The process of breaking down muscles is called catabolism – think catastrophe. The workouts that you'll be performing will cause your body to atrophy initially but don't worry; this catabolic event is soon followed by an anabolic event which results in your body getting stronger and fitter. It's like a dance step – one step backwards, two steps forwards. It's worth remembering, though, that you can only make forward progress if your diet and recovery are optimal.

Exercise Modalities

There are literally hundreds of ways in which you can overload your body to help you improve your fitness and strength. In the workouts later in the book I've selected some of the best methods commonly available, but that's not to say they are the only options. When on deployment, military personnel have to make do with whatever they can find to equip their *ad hoc* gymnasiums, so just because an exercise calls for you to use a barbell doesn't mean that you can't use a heavy rock, sandbag or resistance band instead.

The following is a fairly comprehensive list of strength and cardiovascular training equipment that will crop up during the later workouts. Use whatever you have access to and don't worry if you don't have all the equipment on the list. Remember the motto: improvise, adapt and overcome!

1. **Free weights** – dumbbells and barbells are probably the most traditional and versatile type of equipment for strength training, but if you don't belong to a gym or have a set of weights at home, you can make substitutions very easily by selecting equipment from further down the list. That said, a set of adjustable dumbbells and a barbell will stand you in good stead long after your gym membership would have expired and for far less cost.

2. **Kettlebells** – in effect cannonballs with handles, kettlebells can be swung, lifted or thrown in a variety of ways to challenge your entire body. On the downside, they usually come in fixed weights so you either need a lot of them or need to perform your exercises using different repetition ranges. Kettlebells can be a bit costly, too, but are a good addition to your training arsenal. Many kettlebell

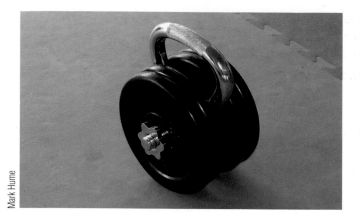

exercises can be performed using dumb-bells, so don't feel that you have to buy one. Where a kettlebell is suggested in any of the workouts within the 12-week programme (Chapter 5), I have endeav-oured to provide you with a dumbbell alternative as well.

Russian soldiers have used kettlebells for the last hundred years to develop fitness and strength.

3. **Sandbags** – cheap and versatile, sandbags offer a viable alternative to free weights. You can make your own or buy a commercial sandbag kit. Sandbags can be used to replicate most barbell exercises and also make less noise when dropped – important if you intend to train at home. Try not to spill sand every-where though as the mess-sergeant may object!

4. **Suspension training equipment** - consisting of nylon straps that can be anchored in doorways or specially fixed eye-bolts, suspension equipment provides the means to make many traditional bodyweight exercises much more demanding. There are a large number of suspension trainers available so do your homework and remember that most expensive does not necessarily mean best. You can also make your own.

5. **Resistance bands** – you can use resistance bands to replicate almost every free weight exercise and also a great many resistance machine exercises too. Light-weight, portable and relatively cheap, resistance bands can be a great at-home option if you don't have space for a free weight set. The main disadvantage with resistance bands is that you don't actually know how much resistance you are using. This makes monitoring and progression of intensity difficult.

6. **Bodyweight exercises** - when push comes to shove, you are your own walking gym. Your body provides the exercise machine and the resistance required to develop a high degree of whole-body fitness. Many strength experts agree that you should only progress to barbell and dumbbell exercises once you have mastered your bodyweight. Needless to say, bodyweight training is a favourite of all branches of the armed forces and is a big part of your coming workouts. Bodyweight exercises can be made more demanding by wearing the civilian equivalent of body armour – a weighted vest. Weighted vests can add a whole new dimension to bodyweight training!

7. **Medicine balls** – these nice but not essential pieces of kit are fun to use and provide an effective way to make many bodyweight exercises more demanding. If you have a medicine ball then feel free to use it, otherwise use a small sandbag, rock, single dumbbell or bag full of books if any of the exercises specify that you need a medicine ball.

8. **Water** – the resistance offered by water can make an excellent training modality, especially if you have an injury that makes traditional strength training impossible. The water supports your bodyweight so you can exercise in relative safety. Deep water running is an excellent alternative to regular cardiovascular exercise if you have a lower limb injury. Consider water training as a viable alternative to your regular workouts if you should be unlucky enough to pick up an injury.

9. **Odd objects** – in Chapter 6, I discuss in depth a variety of strength-training equipment that you can use to develop your muscular performance. In simple terms, anything you can lift is a viable strength-training tool. Your body doesn't know a rock from a kettlebell from a state-of-the-art resistance training machine – it only knows tension. If tension is sufficient, your muscles will get stronger. In time, you'll start to view your entire environment as one great big workout opportunity and then you'll be thinking like a quick-to-improvise member of the military elite!

10. **Treadmills, rowing machines, exercise bikes, etc.** – cardio equipment is a big part of any gym's equipment list but it's by no means essential for your quest to develop military fitness. You can run outside, ride your bike or swim instead. You may need to measure some routes using maps, your car, a bicycle or global positioning (GPS) but you won't need much access to cardio equipment for the workouts. You will, however, need a **skipping rope**. Skipping is an excellent way to warm up and a great cardio conditioning tool and also improves your eye-hand coordination.

Now you have a good grip on basic exercise principles, terminology and types of workout equipment available, let's take a look at some of the different disciplines of training that you will be doing over the coming weeks.

CHAPTER TWO

Getting Physical

The lowdown on muscular endurance, strength and power training ·

Muscle Power

Every movement in your body is powered by muscles. You have very large muscles such as your gluteus maximus (glutes, or butt) and small muscles such as those responsible for opening or closing your eyes. Needless to say, we'll be focusing on your major muscles and developing your body's capacity for work.

Your muscles generate force in one of three ways: as they lengthen, as they shorten and statically. Most exercises involve a shortening phase followed by a lengthening phase, but some may only involve a static phase. Regardless of the method, your muscles generate force; you'll be working to increase your muscular endurance, strength or power.

Military fitness training makes you fit for anything – including boxing and martial arts.

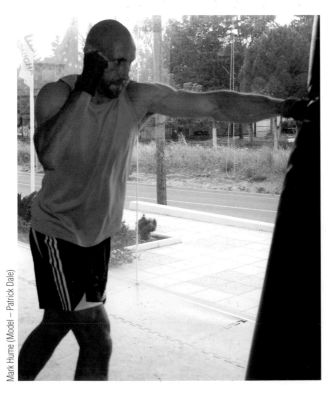

Mark Hume (Model – Patrick Dale)

Muscular endurance describes your ability to perform repeated sub-maximal contractions without suffering undue fatigue. Muscular endurance is an important part of most physical activities and sports and is developed when you perform high-repetition sets with short rests. This floods your muscles with the by-product of anaerobic metabolism, lactic acid. As your muscular endurance improves, your body becomes better able to deal with the build-up of lactic acid and also produces less of it in the first place. Increased muscular endurance essentially makes your body 'fatigue-proof' – essential for almost all physically demanding activities.

Muscular strength describes your ability to generate maximal force for low repetitions. Strength is the result of increased muscle size and an improved ability to recruit more muscle fibres, and is developed by lifting heavy weights for low reps while taking long rests between sets. Strength is important for most sports and also important in the military. For reasons known only to the government, military kit is always twice as heavy as the civilian equivalent! Forces personnel need to be strong to manhandle the equipment necessary so that they can perform their tasks. Strength can also help to injury-proof your body. Strong muscles are less prone to injury and provide support for otherwise unstable and relatively weak joints such as your hips, knees, shoulders and spine.

Muscular power describes when strength is delivered quickly - think kicking a football, lifting a weight quickly, punching, sprinting, jumping or throwing. Power is developed using a type of training called plyometrics and also by performing throwing and Olympic lifting exercises. The Olympic lifts - the snatch, and the clean and jerk - are very technical and beyond the scope of this book, but if you can get qualified tuition they are well worth learning.

What – no Bodybuilding?

The sport and hobby of bodybuilding involves the development of your body's muscles for aesthetic purposes and, although bodybuilding does increase muscular endurance, strength and power, the main focus is muscle hypertrophy or increased muscle cross-sectional size. There is nothing wrong with bodybuilding training but the military athlete needs to function well and not just look good. Don't worry – by following the programmes in this book you will gain muscle size so that you look good in your Speedos on the beach *but*, unlike the typical bodybuilder, your muscles will also be capable of impressive feats of physical prowess. (The programmes do use a few elements of bodybuilding training, but these are tempered with plenty of effective performance-enhancing training methods as well.) Think about it for a second – sprinters and martial artists have some of the best physiques in sports today but they do not train for appearance. These athletes train for *performance* and, as is often the way in nature, form follows function.

The Magnificent Seven

Whatever your fitness level, you will be following one or two strength-training workouts per week. This might not sound like a lot compared to many bodybuilding-style training programmes, but you will be using full body workouts that are built around seven key movement patterns. Many fitness experts make the mistake of getting overly hung up on which muscles are being used rather than how the body actually works. They focus on each individual muscle as though it is possible to isolate it from the rest of the body. This just isn't how your body works. The actions of running, jumping, throwing, carrying, lifting, pushing and pulling use large and complex synergistic muscle groups and so it makes sense, to me at least, that you should train in a similar fashion. Essentially there are seven primary movement patterns that encompass most of your daily physical tasks – hence the Magnificent Seven title to this section.

1. **Squats** – bending your legs and sitting down is one of the most essential movement patterns of all. Getting in and out of your car, sitting on the loo, getting on and off a chair … you perform hundreds of squats every day. Squatting also teaches you to use your legs properly when lifting heavy objects off the ground. Squats are the kings of lower body exercises so expect to be performing plenty of them using weights and just your body. If anyone tells you that squats are bad for your knees, just smile, nod knowingly and then ignore them. This is one of the oldest fitness myths that just refuses to die. With correct technique, squats will actually improve the condition of your knees – far more so than leg extensions or leg presses ever will.

2. **Horizontal pushes** – pushing things away from you is another common movement pattern that you need on a daily basis. For the militarily minded this can include pushing heavy vehicles out of snow drifts or throwing punches during unarmed combat. Horizontal pushing exercises develop your chest, shoulders and triceps and include all forms of press-up and bench press exercises. As mentioned earlier, press-ups are a cornerstone military conditioning exercise, so get used to the idea of doing lots of them. In fact – drop down and give me 20 right now!

3. **Horizontal pulls** – your muscles are arranged in pairs and oppose each other across joints. If one set of muscles becomes overly developed, you can encounter joint problems and muscle function imbalances and increase your risk of joint injury. In the case of horizontal pulling exercises, the muscles between your shoulder blades, your middle trapezius and rhomboids, are the target. It's a little ironic that, in military circles, the press-up is highly regarded but so is good posture. Too many press-ups can actually harm your posture, so it is important to temper all of the horizontal pushing exercises with an equal amount of horizontal pulling. This will keep your shoulders balanced and your posture guard-like and make your drill instructor proud.

4. **Lunges** – lunging is both a movement pattern and a type of exercise that involves a large stepping action to the front, side or rear. While squats are an essential, if static, movement pattern, lunges are much more dynamic and target the muscles involved in locomotive movements such as running. Lunges will also develop your balance and coordination and make a great addition to the Magnificent Seven. Lunges target your thighs and butt so you'll be looking good when/if

Lycra comes back into fashion, and they are a great crossover exercise for running and jumping.

5. **Vertical pushes** – pressing loads above your head is a functional movement that utilizes your shoulders and triceps but is often overlooked in favour of the more glamorous bench press. Not so many years ago, overhead lifting was far more in vogue than bench pressing as a test of upper body strength. Lifting a weight overhead tests your entire body from your legs to your fingertips. In actuality, you are more likely to lift weights above your head than you are to press them away from your chest. You can perform vertical pressing using dumbbells, a barbell, sandbags, kettlebells or resistance bands and you can even perform handstand press-ups. Lifting a weight overhead is sometimes called a military press so expect to be performing a reasonable amount of this particular movement pattern.

6. **Vertical pulls** – as the horizontal pull balances out the horizontal push, this classification of exercise is all about developing equilibrium across muscle groups. It's a case of 'what goes up must come down'. The best exercises that fall into this category are lat pull-downs (which target the latissimus dorsi or upper back muscles) and the far superior but more challenging chin-up and pull-up. Ideally you want to go with chin-ups and pull-ups but, if you aren't quite strong enough yet, lat pull-downs will do for now. You can perform lat pull-downs using a lat pull-down machine at the gym, or by using resistance bands attached to an overhead anchor, but do all you can to progress to chin-ups and pull-ups as soon as possible.

Want a six-pack? Diet is the key!

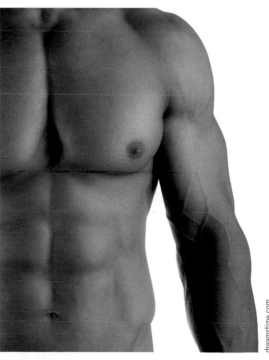

7. **Rotation** – twisting movements are common in life but rarely included in most people's exercise programmes. Throwing a punch, twisting to put your seatbelt on and performing a hip or shoulder throw in self-defence are all examples of rotational movements. The next section on core training will expand on rotation-type exercises but you can be sure that they will feature in all of your strength-training programmes. Rotational exercises will injury-proof your spine, increase your physical performance and also help you towards that elusive and much sought after six-pack!

dreamstime.com

The Core of the Matter

Core is the collective term used by fitness experts to describe your abdominal, waist and lower back muscles. Some of these muscles are on the outside and are readily visible if you are lean enough, while others are deeper and surround your internal organs. These muscles work together to help stabilize your spine and also produce major movements such as bending forwards.

Many people make the mistake of focusing on the muscle at the front of their abdomen – the rectus abdominis. While this muscle is important, it is responsible for just one of the five actions available at your spine. A truly functional midsection is more than just a well-developed six-pack. By developing all of your core muscles equally you will enhance your spine health and function as well as improving your waist aesthetics.

There are five primary movements available at your spine and therefore five classes of exercises that need to be included in your core conditioning workouts.

Movement pattern	Example exercise
1. Flexion of spine	Crunches, reverse crunches, sit-ups
2. Extension of spine	Dorsal raises, back extensions, hip extensions
3. Rotation of spine	Russian twists, cable wood chops, tornado ball
4. Lateral (side) flexion of spine	Side bends, side planks, Saxon side bends
5. Bracing/compression of abdominals	Planks, kneeling on a Swiss ball, dead bugs

By performing exercises that replicate these movement patterns and making sure your core training is multi-dimensional, you will ensure that all the major muscles of your midsection get equal attention and the result will be a better looking, better functioning set of core muscles.

Core Truths, Myths, Mistakes and Outright Lies!

No other area of fitness training and conditioning is surrounded by so many misapprehensions, myths and outright lies as core training. Everyone wants a six-pack but very few seem to be going about their pursuit in a logical way. I'd like to take this opportunity to set the record straight so that you can avoid wasting valuable time on ineffectual workouts.

1. **A well-defined midsection is made in the kitchen.** By this I mean that the chances are, your abdominals (abs) are already pretty impressive but may well be covered in a layer of fat. Lose the blubber and your abs will be revealed. Don't worry – no crazy diets required. Just good, sensible, clean eating combined with

high-intensity exercise will soon carve off the fat and leave you the owner of a highly desirable six-pack.

2. **Targeted exercises cause spot reduction.** Sadly this is not true. Fat is accumulated globally and is used for fuel globally. You need to eat less and exercise more to burn fat and reveal your abs. Endless sets of crunches and sit-ups will not magically reveal your abs. If high reps were the answer to your spot-reduction dreams, wouldn't people who chewed their food a lot have thin faces?

3. **Your abs require more repetitions than other muscle groups.** For some reason, it's a tradition to train your abs with high reps. This myth needs to die! All that happens when you perform high-rep sets is that you delay the onset of fatigue. Fatigue is necessary to trigger an adaptive response. The longer you take to fatigue your muscles, the more time you waste and the less efficient your workout will be. If you can perform more than 20 or so reps of your chosen core exercise you should seek out a more difficult variation or consider adding an external load to make the exercise more challenging.

4. **You should/can train your abs every day.** The muscles of the core are much like the muscles in the rest of your body in that they respond best to intense, relatively brief and infrequent bouts of exercise. You have to give your muscles time to recover from the exercises you expose them to, so daily ab training is another big fat myth.

5. **Heavy core work will make your waist bigger.** The muscles that make up your core are actually quite thin and flat and are very unlikely to grow enough to make your waist look bigger, regardless of the type of core training you do. The burgers, cookies, beers and sweets are far more likely to make your waist look bigger but that's because of fat storage around your middle and not hypertrophy of your core muscles. File this under M for myth.

Belt Up?

While we're on the subject of core conditioning, let's examine the use of weightlifting belts. A weightlifting belt is 10-15 cm (4-6 in) wide and designed to be worn around the waist. Normally made of stiffened nylon or leather, these belts are claimed to support your back, but is this really the case?

You have a natural weight-training belt called your transversus abdominis (TVA for short) which encircles your internal organs. When you contract this muscle, it compresses your abdominal contents and increases intra-abdominal pressure. Intra-abdominal pressure supports your spine from within. Contracting your TVA is simple and involves a process commonly referred to as bracing. To brace your TVA, contract

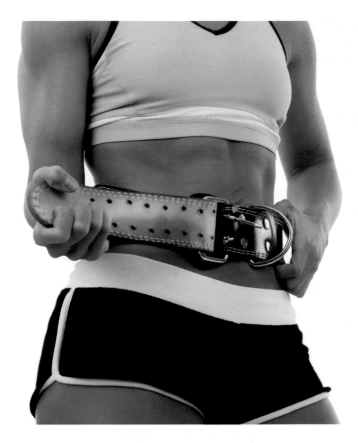

dreamstime.com

Weight-training belts can make your back weaker, not stronger.

your abdominals as though readying yourself for a 'gut punch' and then inhale. You should feel your entire midsection become more solid as intra-abdominal pressure increases.

Wearing a weight belt also increases intra-abdominal pressure, but instead of you pulling your TVA in, your abdominals are pushed out against the belt. There are two problems associated with this: first, you are training your abs to bulge outwards (which is not a good look) and second, if you lift anything heavy when you aren't wearing a belt (for example, picking up your suitcase or heaving your shopping out of your car boot), your abs will bow outwards automatically, as they have been trained to do, but there will be no belt against which to press and produce the necessary intra-abdominal pressure. The result? A reduction in the degree of spinal support and an increased risk of serious lumbar injury.

Many people believe that wearing a weight belt supports your lumbar vertebrae. Sadly this is not the case. Your spine flexes and bends through its entire length, with the exception of your sacrum and coccyx at the very bottom. Wearing a belt simply concentrates all of the force on to a very small area directly above and below your belt. It's like putting a bracket around a pipe and then trying to bend it. All of the force is directed to the points just above and just below the bracket and that is where the pipe will break.

The bottom line is, it is far better to train beltless and rely on your own natural mechanism for creating intra-abdominal pressure than to rely on an external prop that, if not present, will actually result in a weaker lower back than normal. Not wearing a belt means that you have to develop your own core strength to support the efforts of your arms and legs. This means that every exercise you perform while not wearing a belt is a mini-core workout. Belt up? The answer is a resounding 'No'.

If you are a misguided soul who has previously worn a weightlifting belt, please do not ditch it immediately to go cold turkey – this is a quick route to injury. Instead, slowly wean yourself off using your belt by initially using it only for your heaviest sets and then gradually loosening it as you train your TVA to brace and support your spine. This may take weeks and you may find that you initially lose strength but don't worry - you'll soon be strong-backed and beltless and won't have to rely on anything but your core musculature to support your spine.

Core Training Tools

You will need a few things to help you develop your core to the maximum and chances are that you will have easy access to at least a few of these items already.

1. **Stability ball** - a useful piece of kit that can also double as a weight bench, stability balls are between 55 and 75 cm (22 and 30 in) in diameter and can be used for a wide variety of core exercises and drills. Choose a ball that is anti-burst. This doesn't mean that it *won't* burst, just that if it does it will deflate slowly rather than pop like a balloon!

2. **Exercise mat** - a foam exercise mat will make your core work a much more comfortable undertaking and save you having to explain unsightly carpet burns to your spouse! Go for one that is made of closed cell foam so it won't soak up sweat and become smelly. Yoga mats are OK but some users find them a little too thin, although they usually have excellent non-slip qualities.

3. **Ab wheel** - an ab wheel is a small, two-handled wheel that can be used for ab wheel roll-outs (a very effective core exercise). Don't worry if you don't have one of these handy core training tools: you can perform roll-outs using a barbell or stability ball.

You are well on towards building that fitness holy of holies - the six-pack - so now it's time to turn your attention to heart and lung conditioning.

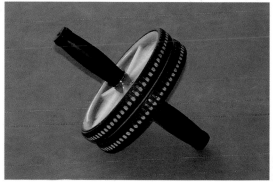

Mark Hume

Ab wheels are old-school but effective

CHAPTER THREE

Combat Cardio

Developing fitness for your heart and lungs

As we have seen, the soldiers of Ancient Greece and Rome had a legendary capacity to cover vast distances on foot prior to engaging and defeating their enemies, and this ability is mirrored by modern infantry units such as the British Paras and Royal Marines. What physical characteristic lies at the core of this ability? The answer is cardiovascular fitness.

Chemical Energy for Life – Adenosine Triphosphate

Your body runs on a very specific fuel molecule called adenosine triphosphate (ATP for short). When ATP is broken down it releases energy, which then is used to power muscular contractions. ATP production can happen in one of two ways – aerobically (meaning in the presence of oxygen), or anaerobically (meaning without oxygen).

ATP – the ultimate renewable energy source!

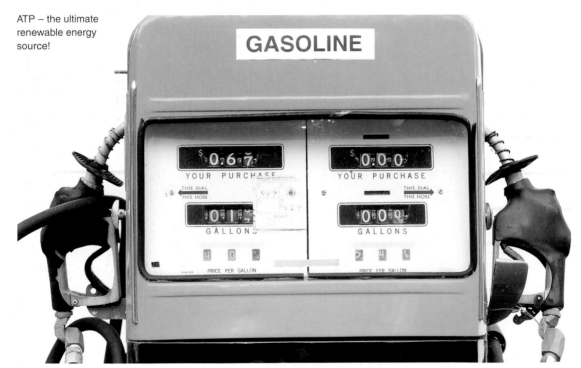

dreamstime.com

With the right kind of training, you can improve your aerobic and anaerobic fitness. If you are finding it difficult to differentiate aerobic and anaerobic activity just remember longer, slower-paced workouts are primarily aerobic while short, intense workouts are primarily anaerobic. Think jogging versus sprinting and walking versus weightlifting.

What is Aerobic Fitness?

Aerobic fitness is the ability of your body to take in, transport and utilize oxygen and is commonly expressed as your VO2 max, which is the maximum volume of oxygen you can effectively use when exercising.

Whenever you perform any kind of aerobic exercise, your muscles demand an increased supply of oxygen and, consequently, your heart and breathing rates increase. Over time, your body becomes better equipped to take in and transport oxygen around your system and, as a result, your work capacity increases. In the long term, your fitness improves because your heart gets bigger, your lung capacity increases and your blood vessels become better able to transport oxygenated blood to, and deoxygenated blood away from, your working muscles.

Aerobic fitness can be developed in a number of ways and you'll get to experience most of them during the training programme that appears later in this book, but common methods include jogging, swimming, running, rowing and cycling. When it comes to choosing your aerobic training modality, weight-bearing activities such as running have a far better real-world carry-over than activities such as aerobic classes. Although all forms of aerobic exercise will increase the conditioning of your heart and lungs, the movement patterns used by each type of aerobic exercise will not necessarily cross over from one modality to another. Fit cyclists do not often run well unless they do some running training as well. Remember the acronym SAID – if you want to become a better runner, then it is running you must do!

You'll also be doing some very specific military-style aerobic training in the form of regular 'yomps'. Yomping is Royal Marine-speak for walking a long way while carrying weight and is a supreme way to develop combat conditioning, strip fat and improve your all-round muscular endurance.

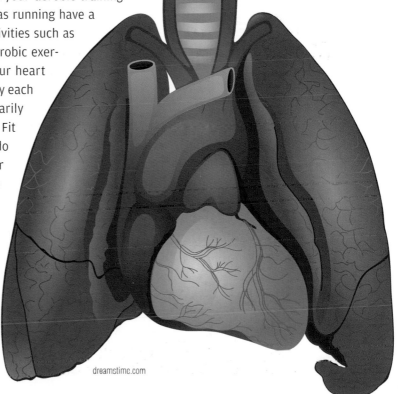

Your heart and lungs ensure that you can take in, transport and utilize oxygen 24/7 and 365 days a year.

dreamstime.com

Monitoring Cardiovascular Exercise Intensity

Cardio training is normally performed for an extended period of time so it's important to choose an exercise intensity that is hard enough to be beneficial but not so hard that it becomes necessary to stop. It is generally accepted that the benefits of aerobic exercise are gained from working at between 60% and 90% of your Maximum Heart Rate (MHR). Many people rely on monitoring their heart rates as an indicator of exercise intensity but this is by no means essential. You can calculate your Heart Rate Training Zone (HRZ) by using these simple formulae:

1. Simple Karvonen Theory

220 – your age in years x 60%

220 – your age in years x 90%

e.g. HRZ for a 40-year-old

220 – 40 = 180 x 60% = 108 bpm (lower end of scale)

220 – 40 = 180 x 90% = 162 bpm (upper end of scale)

2. Heart Rate Reserve

(takes into account elevated fitness levels commonly associated with a low resting heart rate)

220 – age in years – resting heart rate x 60% + resting heart rate

220 – age in years – resting heart rate x 90% + resting heart rate

e.g. HRZ for a 40-year-old with a resting heart rate of 60 bpm

220 – 40 = 180 – 60 = 120 x 60% = 72 + 60 = 132 bpm (lower end of scale)

220 – 40 = 180 – 60 = 120 x 90% = 108 + 60 = 168 bpm (upper end of scale)

Stress Tests for Hardcore Masochists Only!

Alternatively, you can perform a maximal heart rate 'stress test'. The aim of a stress test is to push yourself as hard as possible to generate a maximal heart rate reading. From this figure you would then calculate your heart rate training zone by finding 60% and 90% of your highest reading. Stress tests are, as the name implies, stressful and are not suitable for beginners or those suffering from any kind of exercise contraindication such as high blood pressure.

You can perform a stress test using a flat piece of ground, a rower or any other exercise modality that allows you to work very *very* hard. For this example, we'll use a rowing machine.

After a thorough and appropriate warm-up, row 500 m (550 yards) as fast as you possibly can. Rest for 60 seconds and repeat the row. Towards the end of the second effort, ask your training partner to note your heart rate. Rest one more minute and then perform a final 500 m (550 yard) sprint just to be sure you pushed your heart rate as high as possible. On completion, calculate 60% and 90% of your maximum heart rate.

These numbers represent the lower and upper limits of your HRZ. Going below 60% will essentially negate many of the benefits of exercise as it will be too easy, whereas going above 90% will take you into the anaerobic zone where lactic acid will start to rise and you'll be forced to slow down and stop ... and it hurts too! We'll look more at anaerobic training later in this chapter though, as it's a very useful exercise tool.

To keep an eye on your heart rate while exercising you have a number of options available: you can use a heart rate monitor, you can take your pulse manually at either your wrist (radial pulse) or your neck (carotid pulse) or, if you are using gym-based cardio equipment, you'll find that many machines have built-in hand sensors which measure your heart rate - although some are more accurate than others.

Note, however, that the calculations given above are not infallible - some people don't fit into either of these systems and may find that their HRZ makes exercise either too easy or too hard. Luckily there is an alternative method you can use to monitor the intensity of your cardiovascular workouts ...

The Rate of Perceived Exertion Scale

The Rate of Perceived Exertion Scale (RPE for short) was designed in the 1960s by Gunnar Borg - a Scandinavian exercise expert and cross-country skiing coach. He devised a scale with which to prescribe aerobic exercise to his athletes based on how they felt while training. The original RPE scale went from 6 (absolute rest/inactivity) to 20 (maximum exercise intensity). Why a scale of 6-20? Borg's athletes had an average resting heart rate of 60 bpm and an average maximum heart rate of 200 bpm so he just knocked off a zero. It was found that, with some practice, it was possible to estimate how hard an athlete was working based on how they felt and this corresponded quite accurately to their exercising heart rates. For many people, the classic 6-20 scale is a little awkward to use so it has been simplified and adapted to suit the general exerciser:

1) **Inactive/at rest**
2) **–**
3) **Very light**
4) **Light**
5) **Moderate**
6) **Moderate/heavy**
7) **Heavy**
8) **–**
9) **Very heavy**
10) **Maximum**

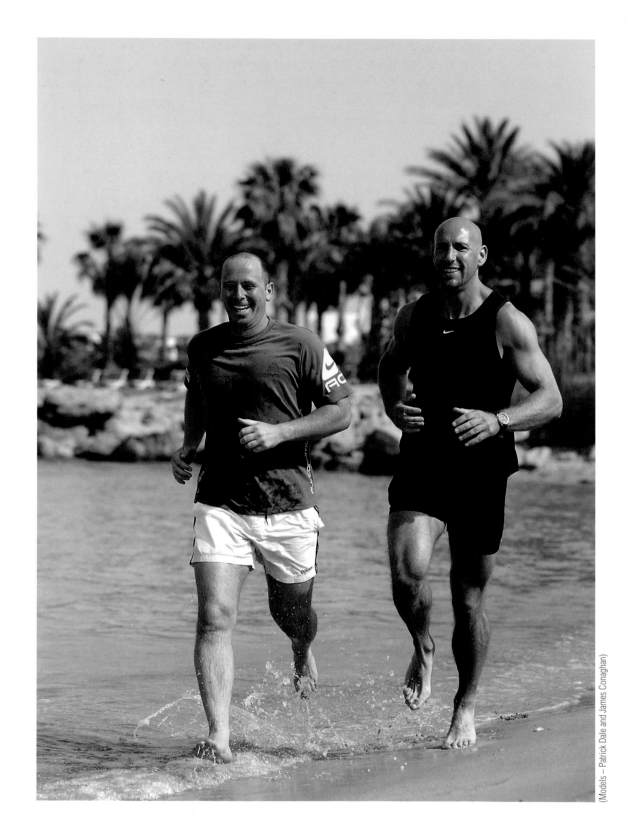

Military Fitness

(Models – Patrick Dale and James Conaghan)

As a general rule of thumb, steady-state aerobic training should be performed at an RPE of 4-7 for maximum benefit. Exercise below this level won't produce much in the way of fitness or health benefits, and above this level will mean approaching the anaerobic zone.

Opposite
The talk test – a simple way to make sure you are working hard enough

Monitoring Breathing and Talking

The final and simplest way to monitor your cardiovascular exercise intensity is by observing your breathing and speech patterns. As your heart rate approaches 60% of maximum, you should find you switch naturally from nose breathing to mouth breathing. In addition, you will need to take a breath every sentence or so as you speak. If you are unable to speak more than a couple of words, you are approaching the upper end of your heart rate training zone, but if you can speak long sentences with no noticeable shortness of breath, you are probably below 60% of your maximum heart rate. By combining RPE with monitoring your breathing and speech rhythms you should have no problem establishing whether you are working hard enough or, in fact, too hard.

Aerobic Training Systems

You will be using a variety of aerobic training methods during the coming weeks to develop your heart and lung fitness. Each method offers advantages and disadvantages, which is why you will be using a mixture of methods rather than relying on just one. As with the strength training you will be performing, there will be one or more methods you take to instantly and probably a few you aren't so keen on. The chances are, the methods you don't like are those that are hardest for you to do and therefore the ones you need to spend more time on - nature is cruel like that!

Long Slow Distance Training

Long slow distance training (LSD for short), describes easy-paced workouts that take place over an extended period of time. LSD is the cornerstone of many runners' training programme. While LSD does increase aerobic fitness and endurance, and can thus be a useful training tool, it does have some disadvantages too.

LONG SLOW DISTANCE TRAINING	
Advantages	**Disadvantages**
'Easy' to perform	Not time efficient
Can aid recovery	Does little to improve high-end fitness
Uses fat as primary fuel	May increase muscle breakdown (catabolism)
Improves low-end fitness and endurance	Teaches you to run a long way slowly!

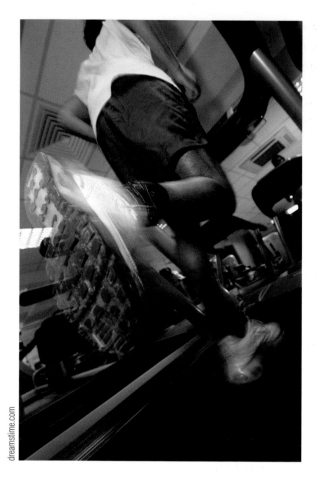

One potential drawback is that LSD workouts tend to be long – marathon runners, for example, often run for two or more hours at a time. The chances are that, unless you are a person of leisure, with no job, partner, hobbies (or life!), such long workouts are going to be prohibitive.

On the subject of marathon runners, when was the last time you saw a long-distance athlete who looked as though they could wrestle an enemy to the ground or manhandle a full ammo box? Most distance runners are generally very slender, lightly muscled and, if truth be told, not all that strong. This is the principle of SAID and natural selection in action. LSD training encourages muscle catabolism. In an effort to make you a more efficient runner, your body sheds muscle weight in an effort to increase your running ability. Shoulder, back, chest and arm muscle mass is detrimental to long-distance running so your body, smart as it is, does everything it can to increase economy and strips you of some of your hard-earned muscle. It's a lot like putting a lighter jockey on a racehorse – less weight for the horse to carry results in a faster horse.

Running on a treadmill is not as effective as running outdoors but is better than the alternative – doing nothing!

Fartlek

Fartlek is an odd word but – trust me on this – it means 'speed play' in Swedish and is a useful training tool. Essentially, fartlek workouts involve running, cycling, rowing or performing any other aerobic exercise at mixed speeds over a pre-set distance or time. In a fartlek workout you alternate between jogging, running, sprinting and walking at random. Increase the pace when you are rested and slow down when you are tired – simple!

FARTLEK	
Advantages	**Disadvantages**
Covers a multitude of fitness 'bases'	Requires discipline
Provides workout variety	Can be a tough workout
Can be customized to individual fitness levels	Improvements in fitness hard to quantify

Why does fartlek require more discipline than LSD? Quite simply, you are your own coach and you must decide when to slow down and when to speed up. It's all too easy to walk for an extra minute's recovery or cut a sprint short because you are feeling tired. You may find that a well-intended fartlek session turns into an easy LSD workout just because you are lacking motivation on that particular day. Fartlek works best when you use physical markers to control your workout: for example, running between lampposts, trees or park benches rather than just arbitrarily increasing and decreasing your pace. Another option is to perform fartlek with a training buddy and take it in turns to choose the next challenge. Fartlek sessions tend to be shorter than LSD sessions, so are a good choice of workout when you are pushed for time.

Fast Continuous Running

The principle of Fast Continuous Running (FCR) can be applied to any aerobic exercise, including running, cycling, swimming and rowing, and it is best thought of as 'race pace' training. Sometimes called 'threshold' or' tempo' running, FCR pace is your fastest sustainable aerobic exercise pace. By sustainable I mean that you *could* go faster but, after a few short, painful minutes, you'd have to slow down and possibly stop. FCR takes you right up to the threshold between aerobic and anaerobic exercise intensities.

FAST CONTINUOUS RUNNING	
Advantages	**Disadvantages**
Short, effective workout	A demanding workout
Improves high-end aerobic fitness	Not suitable for those who are less fit
Triggers a significant energy after-burn	Structurally demanding

FCR workouts tend to be short and sharp because the intensity is so much higher than for LSD and fartlek type workouts. Interestingly, FCR workouts result in greater overall calorie expenditure than LSD workouts, despite being much shorter. This is because of a phenomenon called Excessive Post-Exercise Oxygen Consumption – EPOC for short. EPOC describes how, after a very intense workout, your metabolism remains elevated for hours as it works to rid your body of the waste products built up during your workout, specifically lactic acid and carbon dioxide. EPOC can last up to 24 hours after a hard workout, during which time your calorie expenditure is elevated significantly above baseline. This is great news if you are trying to drop a few pounds of fat. EPOC is like two workouts in one but is not triggered to the same degree by lower-intensity workouts.

A true FCR workout is a mental and physical battle against the effects of lactic acid which will make your muscles and lungs burn and also places increased stress on the structures (muscles, bones, joints, ligaments and tendons) of your body. This means that FCR should be introduced gradually if you are new to higher-intensity exercise, and that it is not suitable for beginners or those carrying injuries.

Interval Training

Interval training can be used to develop either your aerobic or anaerobic fitness, although it is more commonly used for the latter. For the moment, we'll look at the aerobic form; the anaerobic form is discussed later in this chapter.

Aerobic interval training involves running, rowing or cycling at high levels of intensity – up to 90% of your maximum heart rate, and then taking a break before repeating. For example, imagine your best time for a 4-mile (6.4 km) run is 32 minutes, which gives you an average running speed of 8 minutes per mile (or 5 minutes per kilometre). If you were to perform aerobic intervals with a view to increasing your aerobic fitness, you might perform four 1-mile (1.6 km) repeats running at 7 minutes per mile (4.5 minutes per kilometre) with a 5-minute recovery between runs. This means that your cumulative time for 4 miles is now 28 minutes. As you get fitter, you can reduce the amount of time between reps until you are running your mile intervals with virtually no rest in between. Lo and behold, you subsequently beat your best 4-mile time.

Sprinting develops anaerobic fitness and leg power.

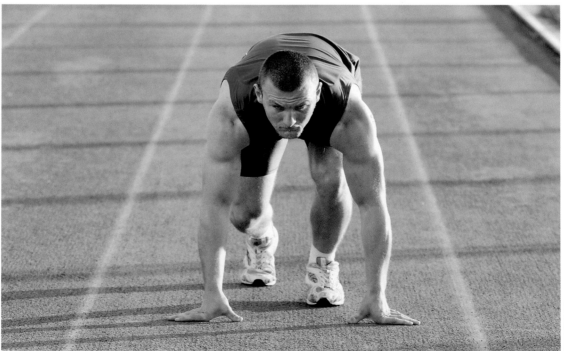

dreamstime.com

Military Fitness

Essentially, aerobic intervals expose you to a higher workload than you could normally sustain but allow you to rest before you get too tired and have to stop.

AEROBIC INTERVAL TRAINING	
Advantages	**Disadvantages**
Short, effective workout	A demanding workout
Improves high-end aerobic fitness	Not suitable for those who are less fit
Improves your running* speed	Structurally demanding
Superior fat-burning workout thanks to EPOC	Requires mental toughness

* Or cycling, swimming or rowing speed, depending on the modality of exercise performed.

What is Anaerobic Fitness?

Anaerobic fitness is the ability to perform high-intensity activity for a relatively short period of time. Most experts agree that 3 minutes is the theoretical upper threshold for anaerobic activity duration, but for most of us mere mortals it's actually more like around 90–120 seconds. Whereas aerobic exercise relies on ATP derived from fat and carbohydrate, anaerobic activity relies purely on carbs. Extracting ATP from carbs is not a very 'clean' process and results in the build-up of fatiguing waste products, specifically lactic acid. When lactic acid levels reach saturation point in your muscles, you have to slow down or stop what you are doing. This is partly because of pain – lactic acid causes that burning sensation associated with hard exercise – but also because lactic acid stops ATP production. Improving your anaerobic fitness means that you must increase your tolerance to the discomfort caused by lactic acid, develop the ability to slow its onset and also train your body to clear it faster.

Why You Need Anaerobic Fitness

Boxers do road work for basic aerobic fitness and weight control. This means, just like Rocky, they head out and run long distances at slow to moderate speeds. However, the sport of boxing is actually more anaerobic than aerobic. Fights are organized into rounds of 3 minutes of action, sometimes fast and furious, other times slower and more controlled, interspersed with 60-second periods of recovery. This type of start/stop activity is anaerobic and the fitness for this kind of endeavour comes from interval and circuit training and not from road work. The road work performed by a boxer develops what is often called an aerobic base, which means a basic level of fitness. Once that is established, higher-intensity workouts will have a much more profound effect on upper end aerobic and anaerobic fitness levels than LSD-type training.

As a Marine, one of the hardest things I ever had to do was not the 48 km (30 mile) forced march or the endurance course – two very aerobic challenges – but Close Quarter Battle or CQB, sometimes called FIBUA or Fighting In Built Up Areas. CQB/FIBUA involves fighting from one building to the next in an urban setting. It's like a never-ending boxing match as you work through building after building in pursuit of the enemy. Climbing through windows, sprinting up stairs, securing prisoners, and then moving on to the next building is a series of maximal-effort bursts of aggressive activity alternated with brief periods of calm in which you reload, regroup and rehydrate. On one particular FIBUA exercise I was so exhausted from clearing house after house after house that, as I tried to leap athletically through a downstairs window, my legs failed and I ended up falling head-first through the thankfully open window and landed on the crouching enemy who was waiting to spring an ambush. While it might have looked like I had been copying a Hollywood action hero, the reality was that I was so exhausted and my limbs so saturated with lactic acid that I was unable to generate much in the way of force or coordination!

Aerobic fitness training alone will not develop your start/stop anaerobic fitness but, ironically, anaerobic fitness will enhance your aerobic energy pathways. Because your heart rate stays elevated during periods of recovery, you get a 'free' aerobic workout when you do an anaerobic one! It's like two workouts in one and every squaddie loves a bargain.

Before you decide never to do an LSD workout again, it's worth mentioning that anaerobic training is very hard and the slower-paced aerobic workouts can provide a pleasant respite from going all-out all the time. Even mighty Marines need to have a bit of rest from time to time!

Anaerobic Training Systems

There are a number of methods that you can use to develop your anaerobic fitness and you'll find most, if not all, will crop up in the programme. You won't like them all, in fact you may actively dislike some of them, but that's because anaerobic training is hard. As the famous German philosopher Friedrich Nietzsche said, 'That which doesn't kill you makes you stronger', or, as military Physical Training Instructors are fond of saying, 'Train harder, fight easier.'

Anaerobic Interval Training

Interval training is *the* classical method for increasing anaerobic fitness and one that will form the cornerstone of many of your coming workouts. As described earlier, interval training is periods of high-intensity work interspersed with periods of low-intensity recovery. The length of the work period and duration of the recovery depend on your current level of fitness, the type of workout you are doing, the modality of exercise you are performing and the training effect you are seeking. The main difference between the aerobic intervals detailed earlier and anaerobic intervals is the speed/intensity of the work periods. Anaerobic intervals must exceed your body's ability to take in, transport and utilize oxygen. This means that although the work periods are shorter, you will need to work harder.

ANAEROBIC INTERVAL TRAINING	
Advantages	Disadvantages
Short, effective workout	A demanding workout
Improves anaerobic and aerobic fitness	Not suitable for those who are less fit
Can be used to develop speed and power	Structurally demanding
Superior fat-burning workout thanks to EPOC	Requires mental toughness

Provided that it takes you above your ability to take in, transport and utilize oxygen anaerobic interval training can involve just about any activity, including running/sprinting, cycling, rowing, punching a heavy bag, skipping, swinging a sledgehammer, performing bodyweight exercises or even lifting weights. Many of the workouts that follow later are 'interval workouts in disguise', as periods of high-intensity activity are broken up with periods of recovery. Circuit training, described later in this chapter, is one such example.

From Japan with Tough Love – Tabata Intervals

It's not often that the reality surrounding an exercise method lives up to the hype, but Tabata intervals are one of the few exceptions. Promising 'improved fitness in just four minutes' may sound like the sort of flannel that you expect to hear on a late-night shopping channel infomercial but the reality is that Tabata intervals work. This training method has been embraced by mixed martial artists, track cyclists, speed skaters, rugby players and the military, so you can be assured that it really is more than hyperbole.

The Tabata Method is named after Dr Izumi Tabata – a sports scientist from the National Institute of Fitness and Sports in Tokyo, Japan. It is a High Intensity Interval Training (HIIT) protocol which has been used successfully by the Japanese Olympic speed-skating team amongst others to improve aerobic and anaerobic conditioning using very brief workouts.

Using eight sets of 20-second maximal-intensity activity coupled with 10-second recovery periods, Dr Tabata achieved some amazing results with his athletes. During his 1997 study, Dr Tabata compared the effects of longer, lower-intensity exercise with bouts of short, very high-intensity exercise. Using his unique interval training method the athletes participating in the study increased their aerobic fitness by

Opposite
Burpees – a great
exercise for circuit
training

14% and anaerobic fitness by 28% in just 8 weeks! It's worth noting that the subjects Dr Tabata used for testing were already accomplished sportsmen and not just beginners, which make this study even more astounding. Still more incredible is the fact that the total actual training time per week was an unbelievable 30 minutes.

Four minutes might not sound like long – you are probably thinking 'just how hard can it be?' The reality is that Tabata intervals may well be the longest minutes of your life! Did I mention that you'll be doing some Tabata-style circuit training as a part of your programme, involving five exercises performed back to back using Tabata protocol? No? Good – I wouldn't want to worry you unnecessarily!

You can apply the Tabata intervals training protocol to a wide number of exercise modalities. Sprinting, squat jumps, kettlebell swings, burpees (more on those later) and rowing are just some of the choices available. The main caveat of Tabata training is that, whatever exercise you select, you perform each set to your absolute maximum ability. No pacing, no saving yourself for a strong finish – perform as much work as possible in the first 20 seconds and then try to maintain that work rate for the remaining intervals. In reality, you probably won't be able to do this, but that's what you have to strive for. Tabata intervals will crop up in the workout programme but, if you are very short of time and have only got 5 or 10 minutes to squeeze in a training session, you now have an excuse-free training method in Tabata intervals.

TABATA INTERVAL TRAINING	
Advantages	**Disadvantages**
Very short and time-efficient workout	Requires access to an accurate timer
Improves aerobic and anaerobic fitness	Tough to perform
Produces significant EPOC	Requires mental discipline

You can manage your Tabata Interval workout by keeping an eye on the sweep hand of a clock or using a stopwatch, but the best way to ensure you stick to the 20 seconds work and 10 seconds rest protocol is to use a programmable timer. There are lots of timer options you can choose from, including software you can run on your laptop or smart phone, watches with built-in timer, or dedicated timer units such as the Gym Boss. I've used them all and, so long as they are simple and reliable, they are all acceptable options. You can always ask a training buddy to keep an eye on the clock while you work out but, as the lactic acid levels climb along with your discomfort, that buddy soon becomes an enemy who, you are convinced, is adding time on to your work periods and taking it off your rests!

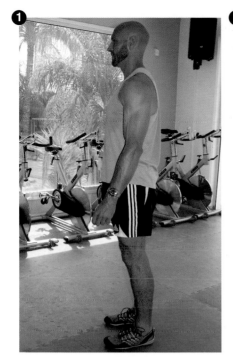

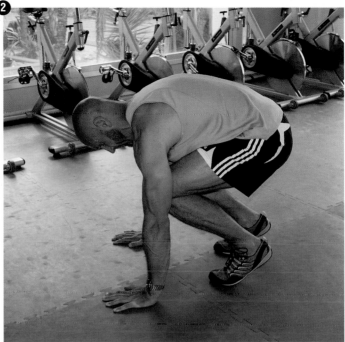

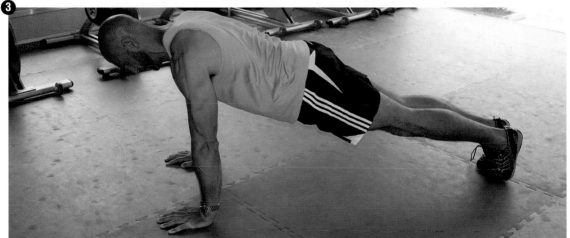

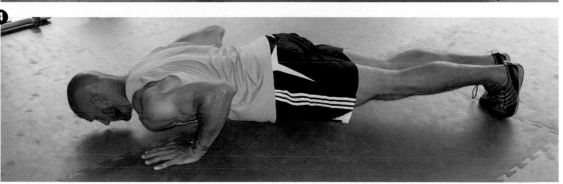

Circuit Training

Circuit training is popular in the military because, in the proverbial nutshell, it works. Circuit training improves aerobic and anaerobic fitness and can also develop muscular strength, power or endurance depending on the exercises used. Circuit training involves performing a series of exercises with little or no rest between them – you only get to rest when you have completed the entire sequence and sometimes not even then (cruel PTIs!).

Circuit training can be repetition or time controlled, by which I mean that you may perform each exercise for a predetermined number of reps or for a set amount of time before moving on to the next station. You'll get a chance to perform both styles of workout – both are equally effective.

Circuit training is an excellent 'go to' form of training when you are short of time and want to cover a multitude of fitness components in one workout. If you ever find that you are struggling to fit in your training and you need a quick fix that gets a lot of work done in the shortest possible time, you could do worse than a few laps of an eight to ten exercise circuit.

CIRCUIT TRAINING	
Advantages	**Disadvantages**
Efficient multi-benefit workout	A demanding workout
Improves anaerobic and aerobic fitness	Not suitable for those who are less fit
Improves muscular strength, endurance and/or power	Exercise technique must be good to minimize risk of injury
Superior fat-burning workout thanks to EPOC	Exercise form can break down through fatigue

Now you know how to develop the lung capacity of a Kenyan marathon runner and the anaerobic fitness of a 400 m hurdler, let's move on to flexibility and mobility, what they are and why you need them.

CHAPTER FOUR

Flexibility and Mobility

It's better to bend like a reed than snap like a tree!

Flexibility is often an overlooked part of many people's fitness routine or, in the case of activities such as yoga, it is the only real focus of a workout. Neither extreme will help you to develop a functional, injury-free, well-aligned body.

Flexibility is developed by performing stretching exercises but, as with all things, there is a right way and a wrong way to go about stretching. Some types of stretches, discussed later, are better suited to your warm-up, while other stretches are more suited to cooling down. Some forms of stretching excite your muscles and nervous system and increase your strength, while other forms of stretching cause your muscles to relax. It's pretty clear then that stretching correctly can enhance your workout experience, while stretching incorrectly can make your workouts less productive. So, like a good recruit, follow these instructions and you'll be on your way to a great workout, a speedy recovery and fewer injuries.

Types of Stretching

There are three main types of stretching which have drastically different effects on your muscles. Choosing the right type of stretching can make the difference between workout success and workout failure. Here are the three types of stretching in order of movement speed:

- Static stretches
- Dynamic stretches
- Ballistic stretches

Static Stretches

Static stretches, as the name implies, involve little or no movement and are designed to maintain or increase your current level of flexibility. To perform a static stretch, slowly extend your limb until you feel tension - called the point of bind - and hold that position. Static stretches held for 10-20 seconds are called maintenance stretches and help prevent your muscles from shortening further, whereas developmental stretches are held for 30-60 seconds and will improve your flexibility. Both types of static stretching cause your muscles to relax and have been shown in studies to reduce the contractile ability of your muscles or, in other words, make you weaker. Don't worry – this weakening is only a temporary effect of static stretching, but it goes to show that static stretching is not an ideal component of a warm-up.

Another downside of static stretches is that they actually cause your body temperature and heart rate to drop and reduce blood flow through your muscles. As the ends of the muscles are stretched away from each other the muscle fibres are pulled together and it is this that reduces blood flow. Static stretches, by their very nature, do not involve any movement and consequently will cause your heart rate to drop. If you've just spent 5 minutes jogging or skipping to get your muscles warm and your heart rate up ready for your workout, and then you spend the next 5 minutes statue-like as you stretch your major muscles, they will now be getting cold. You almost need to warm up again, but who has time for two warm-ups? Another strike against static stretches in warm-ups!

The only exception to the 'no static stretching in a warm-up' principle is if you have a hypertonic (over-tight) muscle that is stopping you from performing an exercise properly. For example, if you have very tight hamstrings, you may find that stretching them statically before a set of squats helps you to avoid rounding your back. This prescriptive use of static stretching is acceptable but also beyond the realms of this book. In most cases, static stretches are best suited to your after-training cool-down, which will be discussed later.

Dynamic Stretches

If static stretches involve no movement, it makes sense that dynamic stretches involve lots of movement. Dynamic stretches don't really look like stretches at all, but the large range of movement employed in this type of stretch means that your muscles are taken through their full range of movement, which helps prepare them for action. Dynamic stretches also mobilize your joints, keep your heart rate elevated, offer a rehearsal opportunity for common exercises such as squats and press-ups and excite your muscles so they are better able to generate maximal force. Dynamic stretches are much better suited to your warm-up than static stretches.

Ballistic Stretches

Ballistic stretches are generally best avoided as they present an increased risk of injury. A ballistic stretch is performed very quickly, for example trying to kick your leg up as high as you can is a ballistic hamstring stretch and flinging your arms back behind you is a ballistic chest stretch. These types of stretches often feature in a pre-sports warm-up because many sports involve ballistic movements. If you are involved in sports such as soccer, kick-boxing or sprinting, ballistic stretching is a necessary evil but, for the rest of us, the benefits of ballistic stretching are outweighed by the increased injury risk.

There is a fine line between dynamic stretches and ballistic stretches. The main thing to remember with dynamic stretching is that you are always in control of the end range of movement for the exercise you are performing whereas, with ballistic stretching, the end range of movement is dependent on the velocity of your limbs. Leg swings performed with control to just short of the point of bind are dynamic, whereas leg swings to full height at speed are ballistic. Thus, although superficially they may appear similar, they are not the same.

Mobility versus Flexibility

Mobility and flexibility are often considered to be the same thing but they are, in fact, two very different fitness components. The term mobility pertains to joints while flexibility pertains to muscles. A good warm-up will address both mobility and flexibility. Dynamic stretching covers both bases in a handful of simple exercises, whereas static stretches only affect your flexibility.

Your joints are mainly synovial in nature, which means they are freely moveable articulations where the ends of your bones are covered in smooth hyaline cartilage and the joint itself is contained within a fibrous capsule. Joints are avascular, meaning they have little or no blood supply. Synovial joints use a special kind of nourishing oil called synovial fluid to keep them healthy and well lubricated. Just as gun oil keeps the moving parts of your M16 rifle working smoothly, synovial fluid makes sure your joints are well lubricated. Synovial fluid is produced in response to joint movements. The more you move, the more fluid is produced. One of the aims of warming up is to increase synovial fluid production. This is done by performing light cardio and dynamic stretches. Static stretches do not enhance synovial fluid production.

Warming Up

Warm-ups prepare your body and mind for exercise. They raise your body temperature, increase the synovial fluid production around your joints, get your muscles to optimum length and provide an opportunity to practise the skills of the workout you are about to perform. The 5-10 minutes spent warming up can make or break your workout. Although it is impossible to prove or disprove that warming up prevents injury – people who have warmed up still get injured after all – it's better to spend a few minutes getting your body ready to train than a few injured months wishing you had!

That said, there are still wrong and right ways to warm up. The former, which we'll call the 'weekend warrior warm-up' as it's the way that many amateur sportsmen get ready for a Saturday afternoon game of football or basketball, goes something like this:

1. Run for 1-2 minutes.
2. Perform static quadriceps (quads) and hamstring stretches.
3. Perform ballistic leg swings.
4. Start playing sport/training at maximum intensity.
5. Play/train badly and/or get injured!

Although such a warm-up is at least better than nothing, for a similar investment in time, you can get a lot more from your pre-training routine and enhance your performance capability as opposed to harming it.

Warming up properly follows a logical sequence of events that will make sure that your body, and indeed your mind, are ready to perform at their best. The stages of a correct warm-up are:

1. Incremental pulse-raising activity
2. Mobility
3. Dynamic flexibility
4. Exercise/activity rehearsal

A cross-trainer warms up your legs and arms.

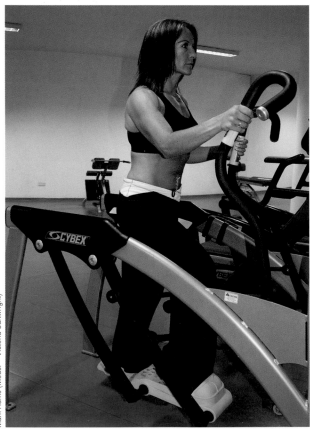

Mark Hume (Model – Victoria Cartwright)

Incremental Pulse-raising Activity

Gradually raising your pulse increases blood flow to your working muscles, raises your core temperature, causes your airways and blood vessels to dilate, increasing oxygen levels in your blood, and helps buffer the fatiguing effects of lactic acid and carbon dioxide. By increasing the intensity of your pulse-raising activity gradually, you make the transition from inactivity to action as smooth and painless as possible. Have you ever noticed how the first few minutes of a run or workout are often the hardest? It's almost as though your lungs can't quite keep pace with your legs! Gradually increasing exercise intensity for the first few minutes of your warm-up prevents this discomfort.

Good examples of pulse-raising activity include jogging, jumping rope, rowing, cycling and using a cross-trainer or stair climber. Using the Rate of Perceived Exertion Scale (RPE) discussed in Chapter 3, you should aim to progress from RPE level 1 to

5/6 over a period of 5-10 minutes. Increase the speed and/or intensity of your pulse-raising activity gradually so that your lungs can keep pace with your legs. You should finish your pulse-raiser slightly out of breath, feeling warm and ready to move on to some more strenuous exercise.

Mobility

Many pulse-raising activities double as joint mobility exercises. Walking, jogging, running, cycling, rowing and stepping mobilize your ankle, knee and hip joints as you raise your temperature. The main disadvantage of cycling, jogging or stepping is, however, that they do little to mobilize your shoulders or spine. Rowing is one of the few pulse-raising activities that cover both the bases of pulse raising and joint mobility. If you choose to warm up by riding a bike, jogging or using a stepper, spend 1-2 minutes mobilizing your major upper body joints prior to exercise.

Jumping rope, aka skipping, is an excellent way to warm up before exercise.

To do this, perform some shoulder shrugs, arm circles, trunk twists, arm bends and neck rolls. About 10 reps of each will get the job done. If you use a rower to warm up you can move straight on to dynamic flexibility. If, however, you use a lower body-dominant form of pulse-raiser, spend a moment on some upper body mobility drills to make sure that your top half is as well prepared for exercise as your bottom half.

Dynamic Flexibility

You now know that dynamic flexibility is the choice of champions for warming up. Dynamic stretches also double as joint mobilizing exercises. Mobilizing your joints twice over may seem like overkill, but synovial fluid is effectively the lifeblood of your joints and, by making sure your joints are well lubricated, you will significantly reduce the amount of exercise-induced wear and tear they experience. This might not seem important now but let me assure you, you'll miss those pain-free, non-creaky joints when they are gone! A few minutes of extra exercise preparation for a decade less joint pain? Count me in!

Perform 10-15 reps of the following dynamic stretches after your incremental pulse-raising activity to ensure that your muscles are ready for your coming workout. Use a controlled tempo and try to increase the range of movement gradually as your set progresses. Concentrate on great posture, good joint alignment and excellent quality of movements to get the most from these simple but effective exercises. Do not perform the exercises forcefully, i.e. in ballistic form, as this may lead to injury.

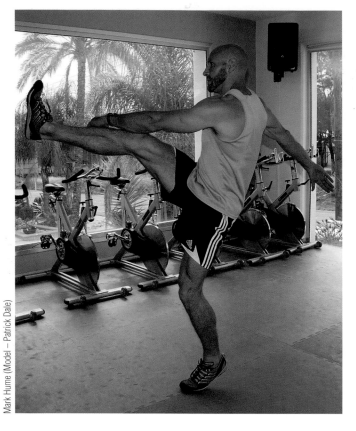

Mark Hume (Model – Patrick Dale)

Dynamic stretch 1 – alternating leg swings. Swing your leg gently forwards as though you were kicking a football. Increase the height of the kicks as you feel your hamstrings begin to loosen up. Reach your opposite hand towards your foot to add a slight twist to mobilize your spine at the same time. Alternate legs by performing a small shuffle step between kicks.

Dynamic stretch 2 – horizontal push and pull. With your arms raised, reach forwards and round your upper back slightly before pulling your arms back and lifting your chest. Alternate pushes and pulls for the desired number of reps. This is a great exercise to prepare your shoulders for press-ups and bench presses and can be combined with a forwards or backwards lunge to also involve the legs.

Alternating leg swings stretch your hamstrings and mobilize your hips.

The horizontal push and pull exercise warms your upper body and simulates performing the bench press and seated row.

❶ 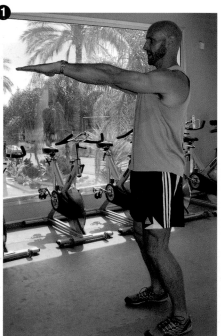 ❷

Mark Hume (Model – Patrick Dale)

Dynamic stretch 3 – squat, reach and twist. This straightforward exercise stretches just about every muscle in your body. Simply bend your knees and squat down and then, as you stand up, reach your arms above your head and rotate your spine slightly so that your upper body is turned to the side. Repeat and twist to the opposite side.

If you only ever perform one dynamic stretch, the squat, reach and twist is the one to choose!

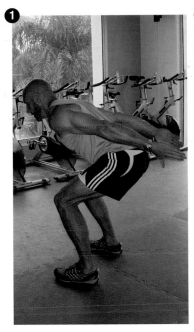
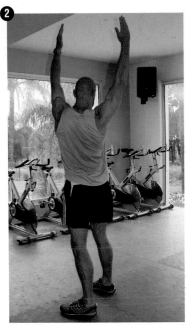

Mark Hume (Model – Patrick Dale)

Dynamic stretch 4 – step overs/duck unders. To really mobilize and stretch your hips, imagine you are standing left side on to a hip-high pole. Step over the imaginary pole and then duck back under it. Perform the desired number of reps and then reverse direction. Perform an equal number of reps on both sides.

Duck unders/step overs prepare your lower body for the demanding exercises to follow.

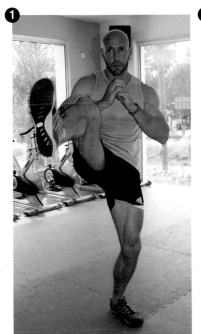
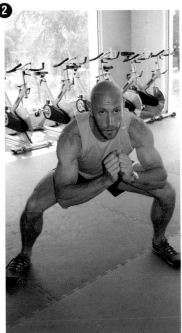
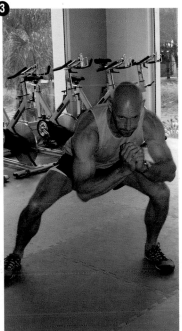

Mark Hume (Model – Patrick Dale)

Exercise/Activity Rehearsal

Now you are warm, your muscles have been stretched and your joints mobilized, it's time to practise a few key elements from your upcoming workout. This might be one or two sub-maximal sets of press-ups or barbell back squats, a couple of half-speed sprints or a few light clean and presses. It all depends on what your workout includes on that particular day. These rehearsals provide you with the opportunity to practise the techniques you'll be performing in your workout and get your mind on the job in hand. Don't go crazy - remember these are preparatory sets and not part of your workout. Do just enough so that you feel you are ready to work out at maximal intensity - you should be itching to get started after a good warm-up!

How Long Should a Warm-up Be?

This question, valid as it is, cannot really be answered. There are a number of factors that need to be considered which dictate the length of your warm-up. Consider these factors and then warm up accordingly. Remember that, at the end of your warm-up, you should feel you are fully prepared and energized and not feel tired or cold and tight.

Consideration	Effect
Inactive for long period prior to workout	Longer warm-up required
Low temperature of surroundings	Longer warm-up required
Intense workout to follow	Longer warm-up required
Age	Older exercisers benefit from longer warm-ups
Joint pain or muscle stiffness	Longer warm-up required
Low-intensity workout to follow	Shorter warm-up required
Time of day	Early morning workouts benefit from longer warm-ups

Warm-ups should be long enough to get the job done but no longer than necessary. On average, allow 5-15 minutes for your warm-up. It's better to do a couple of minutes too long than a couple of minutes too short and remember - time spent warming up might save you months of inactivity because of an otherwise avoidable injury.

Cooling Down

So, your workout is finished, and you are exhausted and hungry. Probably the last thing you want to do is spend another 5-10 minutes performing yet more exercise - after all, you'll get cooler by doing nothing, right? The problem is that if you just come to an abrupt halt after a workout, all of the metabolic waste products produced during your workout are still in your muscles, and failing to flush them out can result in hampered post-exercise recovery and sore muscles tomorrow. A few minutes spent returning to your original pre-exercise state – called homeostasis – means you'll recover faster and be able to train harder, sooner.

There are two phases to cooling down:

1. Incremental pulse-lowering activity
2. Static stretches

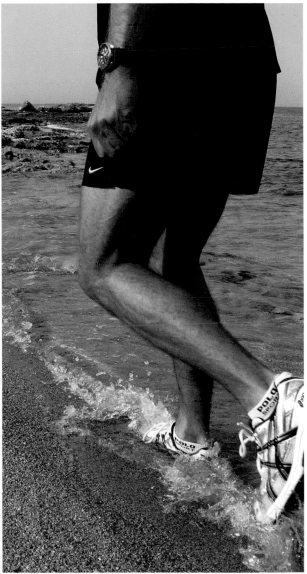

To cool down effectively, reduce your exercise intensity over a few minutes.

Incremental Pulse-lowering Activity

The aim of the incremental pulse-lowering is to promote venous return and help supply your hard-worked muscles with freshly re-oxygenated blood. When you work out, blood 'pools' within your working muscles and, with it, the waste products of metabolism accumulate. Flushing your muscles through with freshly oxygenated blood helps clear these metabolic remnants away and promotes recovery. Pulse-lowering merely requires the reversal of the pulse-raiser performed in your warm-up – perform some cardio at a reasonable level of intensity and then reduce your speed over 3-5 minutes. You should finish your pulse-lowering with your breathing approaching normal and feeling ready to do some stretching. You can use any form of cardio for your cool-down but avoid activities you find demanding.

Static Stretches

The dynamic stretches performed in the warm-up are great at preparing your muscles for exercise but not so good for improving or maintaining your flexibility. The better choice of stretch for your cool-down is static stretches, as described at the start of this chapter. As mentioned, these can be either maintenance (short duration to main-tain flexibility) or developmental (longer

(Model – Patrick Da e)

duration to improve flexibility) in form. Your cool-down may contain one or both types of stretching depending on your current flexibility requirements.

When it comes to stretching duration, you will know which muscles feel tight and which ones don't. Spend longer on the tight muscles and less time on the looser ones.

Adaptive Shortening – When Exercise Goes Bad

The effects of exercise are very specific. Remember the SAID principle – Specific Adaptations to Imposed Demands. This simply means that your muscles adapt to the stresses put on them. If the exercises you perform use a short or restricted range of movement then your muscles will adapt to that stimulus. If you run with a short length stride, the muscles responsible will shorten. If you perform press-ups then your chest muscles will shorten according to the range of movement you use. In essence, short-range movements used in most common exercises can make your muscles shorter – this is adaptive shortening.

Stretching after a workout can help to reset your muscles and return them to their original resting length, or even enhance your flexibility by encouraging your muscles to rest in a new, lengthened position. The static stretching used in the cool-down also helps to relax your muscles and rebalance your nervous system – both essential for recovery after exercise. Get the most from your stretches by following the tips below.

Seven Tips for Better Stretching

1. Only stretch your muscles when they are warm – stretching cold muscles may lead to injury.
2. Do not bounce! Bouncing when stretching is dangerous and can result in injury.
3. Stay relaxed when stretching – do not let your shoulders, jaw, neck or hands tense up as this will reduce the effectiveness of your stretching.
4. Breathe! Exhale as you relax into a stretch. Holding your breath will only impair your stretching.
5. If you are really inflexible, consider stretching every day – possibly twice or more for particularly stiff muscles. If it's taken you years to stiffen up, it'll take more than a few minutes a week to make you flexible again!
6. If you find it difficult to find the time to stretch after your workout – maybe because you are hungry or in a rush to get to work – just perform a few maintenance stretches after exercising and then have a proper stretch when it's more convenient, e.g. when watching the TV at the end of your day.
7. Never force a stretch – if you feel any burning, or your muscles are shaking uncontrollably, you are overdoing it, so back off before you hurt yourself.

Your Personal Stretching Prescription

To save you from having to design your own cool-down, just perform the following stretches after each and every workout, but only once you have completed your pulse-lowering activity. Hold the stretches for as long as you deem necessary based on your flexibility and remember to spend longer on the muscles that feel tightest.

1. Standing calf stretch. Stand arms' length from a wall or post and place your hands out at shoulder level. Step your right leg back and bend your left knee. Press your right heel into the floor, ensuring that your ankle, knee and hip are aligned and your right foot is pointing straight at the wall. Keep your head and chest up for the duration of the stretch. Change legs and then repeat.

2. Standing quad stretch. Perform this stretch next to a wall or post if you need help with balance. Bend your right leg behind you and grasp around your ankle with your right hand. Point your right knee down at the floor and keep your legs together. Pull your right foot towards your butt. Hold this position while maintaining an upright torso. On completion, change legs and then repeat.

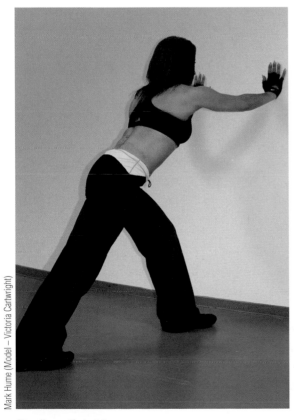

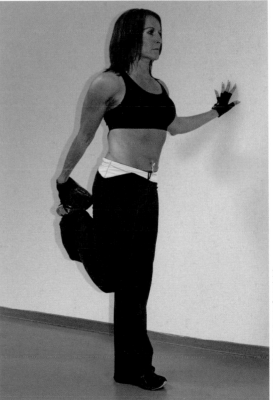

Standing calf stretch

Standing quad stretch

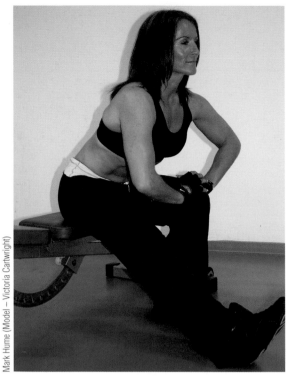

Mark Hume (Model – Victoria Cartwright)

Seated hamstring
stretch

3. Seated hamstring stretch. Sit on a bench or chair with your legs bent and feet flat on the floor. Extend one leg in front of you and place your heel on the floor with your toes pointing up towards the ceiling. Place your hands on your bent knee and then, keeping your chest lifted, lean forwards from your hips. Try not to let your lower back round over as you lean forwards. Hold for the desired duration and then change legs.

4. Kneeling hip flexor stretch. Kneel down on the floor and then take a large step forwards so that your front shin is vertical and your rear leg is extended behind you, knee resting on the floor. Keep your body upright. Relax and sink your hips down towards the floor. Slide your rear leg further back if necessary. Place your hands on your front thigh and hold this position for the required duration. Come out of the stretch slowly, change legs and repeat.

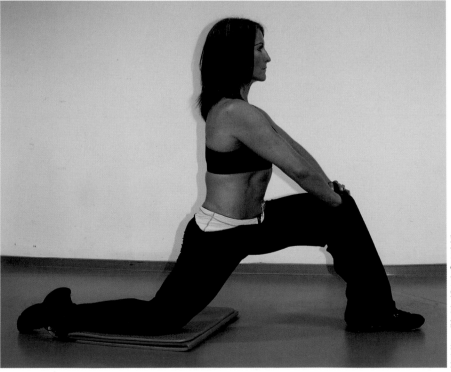

Kneeling hip flexor
stretch

Mark Hume (Model – Victoria Cartwright)

5. Seated groin stretch. Sit on the floor with the soles of your feet together and your legs bent. Draw your feet as close as possible to your groin. Wrap your hands around your ankles and place your elbows on your legs. Use your arms to push your knees gently down towards the floor. This stretch is more effective if you remove your shoes. Try not to let your lower back round excessively when performing this exercise.

6. Prone-lying ab stretch. Lie on your front with your hands below your shoulders and your forehead resting on the floor. Gently lift your head, chest and shoulders off the floor while simultaneously pushing with your arms. Keep your arms close to your ribs and your chin tucked in. Keep your hips on the floor and your legs straight throughout this stretch.

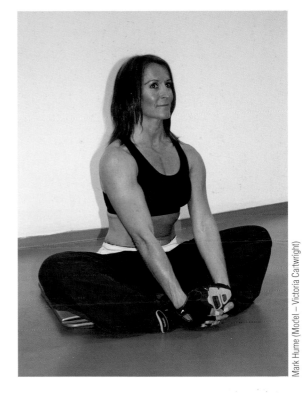

Seated groin stretch

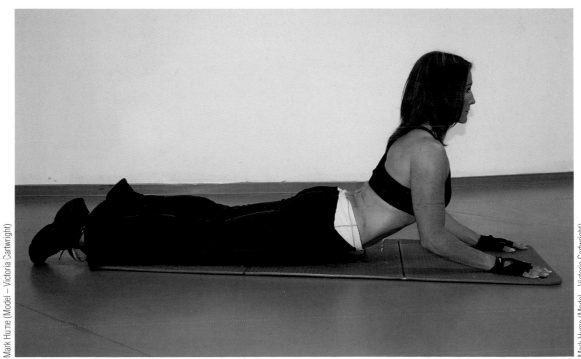

Prone-lying ab stretch

7. Supine-lying glute stretch with spinal twist. Lie on your back with your legs straight and your hands by your sides. Bend your right leg and place your foot next to your left knee. Put your left arm on the floor at shoulder height and reach your left arm across your body, grasping the outside of your right knee. Roll your lower body to the left, keeping your right arm flat on the floor. Hold this position for the desired duration before slowly returning to the centre and then repeat the stretch on the other side.

Supine-lying glute/spine stretch

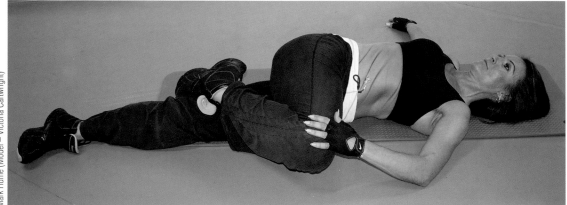

Mark Hume (Model – Victoria Cartwright)

8. Doorway chest stretch. Stand in an open doorway and place your forearms on the vertical door frames. Your elbows should be level with your shoulders and your arms bent to 90 degrees. Adopt a staggered stance and then lean your chest between your arms to stretch your chest and shoulders. Hold this position and then slowly ease out of the stretch. If you don't have a doorway available, perform this stretch one arm at a time against any vertical support such as the corner of a wall, a tree or a lamppost.

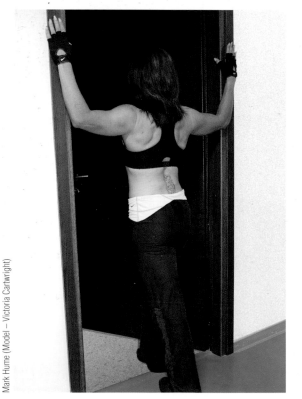

Mark Hume (Model – Victoria Cartwright)

Doorway chest stretch

9. Standing lat stretch. Grasp a sturdy waist-high handhold with your left hand. Move your feet backwards and lean forwards until your upper body is parallel to the floor and your arm is fully extended. Lean your body towards your left arm to deepen the stretch in your lats while also leaning back to stretch your shoulders. Hold this position for the desired duration and then change sides.

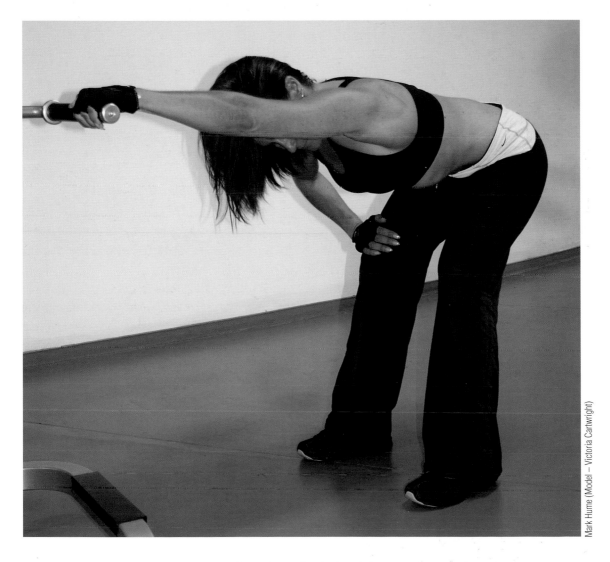

Mark Hume (Model – Victoria Cartwright)

Standing lat stretch

Remember the wise words of the Royal Marines' Physical Training Instructors: 'If you don't have time to warm up and cool down properly, you don't have time to exercise!' Skimping on these vital elements of your workout can hamper your progress and actually reduce your fitness. Make sure you allow sufficient time for your warm-up and cool-down. Consider this a 'standing order', from which deviation may result in reduced recovery and/or injury.

CHAPTER FIVE

Your 12-week Military Fitness Training Plan

A plan for total fitness and strength

This training plan is designed to be progressive and encompasses all of the fitness components necessary to develop military fitness. Each workout can be scaled to suit your individual fitness needs by adding or subtracting volume or raising or lowering intensity. The workouts should be challenging, but not impossible. Wherever possible, you will be provided with options so that you can perform the workouts irrespective of where you train or what equipment you have access to and Chapter 6 provides information on how you can acquire, make or otherwise get your hands on cheap equipment alternatives.

The plan consists of three 4-week blocks which include numerous repeating elements so that you can measure your performance and see the fruits of your labours. There are also monthly progress tests in the form of the Military Fitness Physical Training Assessment or MFPTA for short. Treat the tests as a competition against yourself. If a test requires you to perform a maximum repetition set of pull-ups, make sure you don't drop off that bar until you are absolutely spent. Keep a record of your MFPTA test scores on the table provided on p. 71.

Wherever possible, try to do the workouts on the allotted days but if, because of work or family commitments, you need to change your training days then please do – better that than missing a workout altogether. Try to avoid performing a boot run on the day immediately before or after a yomp as this may cause your run or yomp to suffer.

Programme Overview

	Monday	Tuesday	Wednesday	Thursday	Friday	Saturday	Sunday
Week 1	MFPTA	Boot run 10 mins	Strength training 1	Rest	Troop phyz 1	Yomp 60 mins	Rest
Week 2	Troop phyz 2	Boot run 11 mins	Strength training 1	Rest	Troop phyz 3	Yomp 65 mins	Rest
Week 3	Troop phyz 4	Boot run 12 mins	Strength training 1	Rest	Troop phyz 5	Yomp 70 mins	Rest
Week 4	Troop phyz 6	Boot run 13 mins	Strength training 1	Rest	Troop phyz 7	Yomp 75 mins	Rest
Week 5	MFPTA	Boot run 14 mins	Strength training 2	Rest	Troop phyz 8	Yomp 80 mins	Rest
Week 6	Troop phyz 9	Boot run 15 mins	Strength training 2	Rest	Troop phyz 10	Yomp 85 mins	Rest
Week 7	Troop phyz 1	Boot run 16 mins	Strength training 2	Rest	Troop phyz 2	Yomp 90 mins	Rest
Week 8	Troop phyz 3	Boot run 17 mins	Strength training 2	Rest	Troop phyz 4	Yomp 95 mins	Rest
Week 9	MFPTA	Boot run 18 mins	Strength training 3	Rest	Troop phyz 5	Yomp 100 mins	Rest
Week 10	Troop phyz 6	Boot run 19 mins	Strength training 3	Rest	Troop phyz 7	Yomp 110 mins	Rest
Week 11	Troop phyz 8	Boot run 20 mins	Strength training 3	Rest	Troop phyz 9	Yomp 120 mins	Rest
Week 12	Troop phyz 10	Boot run 20 mins	Strength training 3	Rest	MFPTA	Yomp 120 mins	Rest

Troop Phyz

There are 10 troop phyz (Marine-speak for troop physical training) workouts and each one is repeated twice during the 12-week programme. These workouts are broad in variety, modality and intensity but, regardless of which of the 10 workouts you are performing, you must endeavour to work at the highest level that you can. The troop phyz workouts are short, sharp and simple and, in most cases, can be performed almost anywhere you can find some space. The main aim of the troop phyz workouts is to develop your muscular endurance and anaerobic conditioning but, as you'll see, this is not always the case. The slightly chaotic design of the workouts is intentional – in the military, no two days are the same and, consequently, the programmes in the workout reflect this.

Boot Runs

Despite the name, you don't have to wear boots for these workouts, but if you are using this programme to help you prepare for a life in the armed forces, it's not a bad idea. Boot runs are out-and-back runs where you run easily in one direction and then try to run back to your start point as fast as possible. The runs get longer each week as you increase the length of the outward journey. The time designation refers to the length of the outward run. On reaching the turnaround point, stop, catch your breath, compose yourself – a favourite expression of military PTIs – and then head back the way you came as fast as you can. You should aim to complete each boot run feeling as though you couldn't have run any quicker, even if you wanted to.

If you are an accomplished runner, feel free to increase the length of the boot runs; alternatively, if running is not one of your strengths, reduce the length. *However*, if you do alter the length of the boot run, make sure you still adhere to the progressive nature of this workout by increasing the length of the outward journey every week. Most importantly, do not add so much distance to your boot runs that you end up too tired to complete the rest of the week's training.

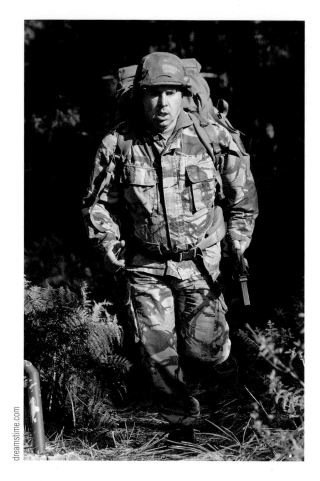

Boots and combat gear optional!

Strength Training

Strength is important, but big bodybuilder-sized muscles are about 'as much use as a chocolate teapot', to use another favourite armed forces expression. Your strength workouts will focus on developing functional whole-body strength and not pumping up your muscles for the beach. The strength-training workouts are short, simple and demanding and focus on the Magnificent Seven movement patterns described in Chapter 2. Instructions on how to perform each exercise are provided but if you are unsure about any exercise techniques, seek expert advice from a qualified personal trainer or gym instructor. Poor technique may lead to injury so, if in doubt, get help. The workouts change slightly every four weeks to provide you with exercise variety and to illustrate that there are plenty of ways to skin the proverbial cat when it comes to strength training. There is also an option for increasing strength-training frequency from once a week to twice – handy if you want to pack on some muscle.

Yomp

Yomping is, as you know by now, Marine-speak for walking a long way over mixed terrain while carrying a heavy load. Yomping requires and develops aerobic fitness, leg strength and mental fortitude. For your yomps you will need a rucksack or, if you prefer a more gym-friendly and high-tech approach, a weighted vest. As yomping will probably be very new to you, be initially conservative with the weight you load into your backpack or weighted vest. Start off with around 10% of your bodyweight and increase gradually from there. Because of the extra load you will be carrying and therefore placing on your feet, it is important to wear supportive shoes or preferably boots when yomping. A yomp is not an easy-paced stroll - far from it. Aim to cover the ground as quickly as possible without actually breaking into a run. Lean forwards slightly from the hips, swing your arms purposefully and stride out. The numerical notations in the programme refer to the total duration of your yomps in minutes. Adjust the duration to suit your current level of fitness but, as with the boot runs, make sure that you increase the duration on a week-by-week basis, likewise the amount of weight in your backpack/weighted vest by ½–1 kg (1–2 lb) per week.

While you can perform your yomping on an indoor treadmill, you will gain far more benefit and enjoyment if you grab your rucksack or weight vest and head out into your local area. Use your yomps as an opportunity to explore, enjoy some countryside and maybe, as any good squaddie would, end up at a countryside pub for a well-deserved pint at the end!

Feel free to carry supplies for consumption during your yomp. Details on exercise nutrition can be found in Chapter 7.

A heavily loaded backpack makes yomping more challenging, realistic and beneficial.

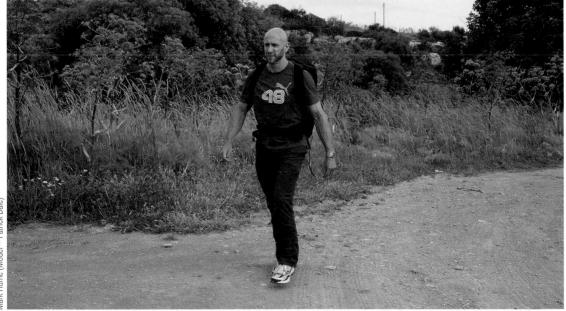

Mark Hume (Model – Patrick Dale)

Rest

Rest is a vital but often overlooked aspect of anyone's training. While a good work ethic might suggest that more training is better, it's important to remember that rest days and when you are sleeping are the times when your body makes its adaptations to exercise which result in your increases in fitness and strength. Treat each rest day as exactly that. For some reason I never understood, Royal Marines called resting up Egyptian PT. Enjoy your rest days, engage in some hardcore Egyptian PT and don't be tempted to add any more training volume to the programme. Just like the basic military training followed by recruits the world over, you are working towards a definite goal where, at the end of the 12 weeks, your fitness will peak. The only way to achieve such a high peak in fitness is to follow a logical and progressive plan. Resting is a vital part of that plan, so train hard and then rest hard.

What Next?

Once you have completed the 12-week plan in its entirety, take a week off training and then start again. Reduce your workout intensity and duration slightly and then proceed to build up to a new peak of fitness – think five steps forwards, one step back. Once you have completed the programme, feel free to design your own troop phyz workouts and strength-training sessions but, for your first run through, stick with the workouts that have been provided for you and follow the instructions to the letter. Once you have graduated from training and completed your first cycle of 12 weeks, you can consider yourself promoted and therefore qualified to make a few changes to the plan!

Notes on Exercise Technique

Precision

To get the most from your workouts and minimize your risk of injury, make sure you perform each and every exercise with military precision and perfect form. Study the pictures and text and make sure you know how to do each exercise properly. If any of the exercises are new, spend a few minutes before each workout familiarizing yourself with the intricacies of the exercises by performing some lightweight practice sets. Only once you are proficient with the exercises should you start loading up and going eyeballs out! Remember – you cannot train if you are injured and pulled muscles are your mortal, personal enemy. It is often better to retreat and regroup than bash your head against the proverbial brick wall. Train hard but also train smart.

Scaling the Workouts

The workouts that follow are designed to be challenging but that doesn't mean that you can't adapt them to suit your own individual fitness levels. If appropriate, reduce the number of reps, increase the rest periods, reduce the weights, perform fewer sets or use a less demanding but similar exercise. Any trainer can exercise you to within an inch of exhaustion in a matter of minutes but a *good* trainer gets you very close to your physical limit and manipulates the training variables so you can complete your workout – albeit only just! Push yourself but always make sure you finish your workouts – failure is not an option. Over time, as your fitness increases, work your way up to performing the workouts as they are prescribed. This may take weeks, months or longer but that's OK – every improvement, no matter how small, is cause for celebration.

If you want to make any of the workouts more demanding, just strap on a weighted vest, increase the reps, perform more sets, reduce the rest periods or choose more demanding but similar versions of the prescribed exercises. Use the workouts as templates or suggestions rather than treating them as set-in-stone commandments.

Where to Work Out

As mentioned, you can perform most if not all of the following workouts in most gyms. Chances are, however, that you won't actually need much of the equipment that your membership fees are paying for. This begs the question: do you really need to join a gym to get militarily fit? I own a gym and seldom work out there! And on the rare occasions I do train at my gym I only use a very small amount of the kit available and, in actuality, need the space more than I need the equipment it contains. As mentioned, in the next chapter I will outline some low-tech but highly effective exercise equipment options that you can use to create your own home gym set-up for less than your annual gym membership.

Training on your home turf actually offers some real advantages:

- Your home gym is always open – you can train at any time you like.
- No queues for equipment – essential when you are performing circuit training or a workout 'against the clock'.
- You'll avoid the usual airborne bugs that are so prevalent in gyms and spread through the air conditioning systems. Why people choose to exercise when they have a cold I really can't say, but you can guarantee that germs and viruses travel like wildfire via air conditioning.
- No distractions. People will want to ask you about the training routine you are doing. If this happens you have two options – stop and talk to them, which may compromise your workout, or don't stop, which may make you appear rude. Either way, a lack of distractions will only add to the quality of your workouts.
- You can choose what music you want to listen to while you exercise – death metal, 80s synth pop or gangster rap – no matter how offensive your music choices might be, you can play what you like as loud as you like!
- You'll save money. Once your home gym is up and running there are no ongoing costs. The rest of your family can work out as well at no extra cost.

That said, some of the workouts that follow are actually better suited to the great outdoors. In terms of venue, you may have to do a bit of reconnaissance around your local area to find appropriate training venues, but after a while you will probably start viewing your surroundings as one big potential gym. The monkey bars at the local park morph into a virtually perfect location for pull-ups and dips; the steep hill at the end of your road will be perfect for hill sprint intervals; the disused patch of land would make an ideal venue for some sledgehammer conditioning drills; the big rock at the bottom of your garden will make an excellent strength-training tool. I'm not anti-gyms at all but you can develop a very high level of fitness without ever setting foot in a chromed and mirrored fitness palace simply by, as any good soldier would, exploiting your surroundings.

When to Work Out

There are a number of opinions as to the best time to exercise. Various experts have proposed one time or another that is, they say, the time at which your workouts will be safest and most productive. Joint mobility, hormonal secretions, body temperature and even your height changes throughout the day so, these boffins say, you should take all this information into account when deciding when to train. As it turns out, the general consensus of opinion as to when you should exercise is around 4 p.m.

This is all well and good in a perfect world, but what if you can only train late at night once the kids are asleep, or early in the morning because that's the only time you have free? Does this mean that exercising at any time other than 4 p.m. is a waste of time or potentially harmful? Of course not! The best time for you to exercise is the time that fits seamlessly into your daily schedule. Maybe 4 p.m. is the ideal time, but if you're stuck at work, picking the kids up from school or otherwise engaged, this little factoid is completely irrelevant. Train at a time that suits you. I've trained at 5 a.m., 4 p.m. and even midnight, depending on what my schedule allows. I can honestly say that, in terms of results, I've noticed no difference from one workout time to the next. The only thing I would say is that if you are training very early in the morning you should consider warming up for a little longer than normal as your body may not be as mobile as usual.

Right then – it's time for less talking and more action! On to the workouts …

Military Fitness Physical Training Assessment

Equipment: exercise mat, stopwatch, pull-up bar, marker cones, measuring tape.
Duration: 20-30 minutes plus warm-up and cool-down.
Purpose: to assess current levels of fitness.
Method: after you have warmed up, perform each of the following exercises to the best of your ability. Record your results in the chart supplied below and endeavour to equal or beat your scores on subsequent tests.

Test one - Maximum reps of press-ups - unlimited time.

Test two - Maximum reps of pull-ups - unlimited time.

(Option - perform body rows if you are unable to perform pull-ups.)

Test three - Maximum reps of sit-ups - 60 seconds.

Test four - 300 m (330 yard) run.

Test five - Maximum number of burpees - 180 seconds.

Take 5 minutes between tests, or longer if necessary. For press-ups and pull-ups, continue until you are unable to perform another rep in good form. For all other tests, use a stopwatch. You may find it beneficial to have someone do the timing for you.

Test	Date	Press-ups	Pull-ups	Sit-ups	300 m run	Burpees
1						
2						
3						
4						
5						
6						
7						
8						
9						
10						

EXERCISE DESCRIPTIONS

Test one – press-ups

While everyone *thinks* they know how to do a proper military-style press-up, the reality is quite different. I've trained literally hundreds of clients and almost all of them, including the very fit ones, perform press-ups with very shabby technique. Perform press-ups properly or get out of my gym soldier-boy!

- Bend down and place your hands on the floor, shoulder-width apart. Point your fingers forwards.
- With your arms straight, walk your feet back into the press-up position.
- Check that your heels, hips and shoulders form a straight line.
- Keep your core muscles tight and your neck long - tuck your chin in slightly.
- Bend your elbows and, keeping your arms tucked into your ribs, lower your chest to within 2-3 cm (an inch) of the floor.

- Push back up and return to the starting position.
- If full press-ups are too challenging, bend your legs and place your knees on the floor. This is the three-quarter press-up.

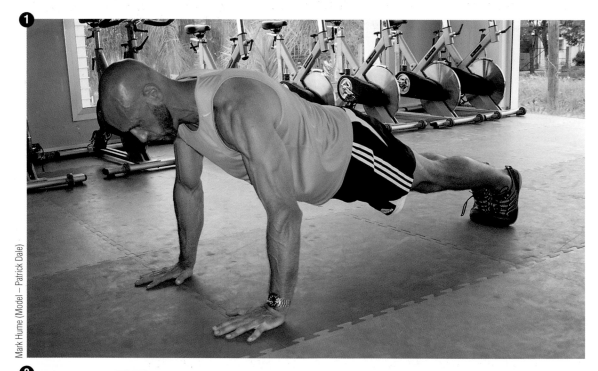

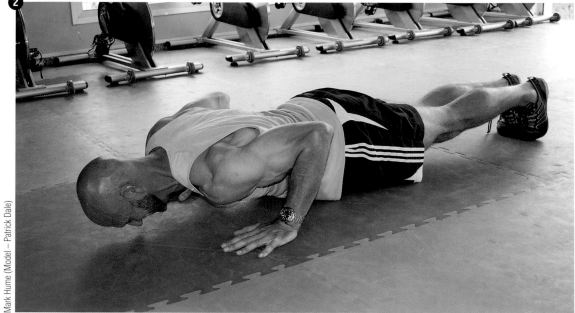

Perform your press-ups with perfect form!

Test two – pull-ups

One of the more challenging bodyweight exercises, pull-ups target your upper back, biceps and core muscles. You'll need a sturdy overhead bar for this exercise that allows you to hang full-stretch without your feet touching the floor.

- Grasp an overhead bar with a slightly wider than shoulder-width overhand grip.
- Hang at full stretch with your arms and legs extended - this is called the dead hang position.
- Pull strongly with your arms and lift your chin up and over the bar.
- Slowly lower to the starting position and repeat.

Test two (option) – body rows

If you are unable to perform pull-ups, you can perform body rows instead. This exercise uses similar muscles but the inclined position of your body reduces the effect of gravity somewhat.

- Adjust the bar on a Smith machine or squat rack to hip-height.
- Sit beneath the bar and grasp it with an overhand shoulder-width grip.
- Extend your legs and lift your butt off the floor - your heels, hips and shoulders should form a straight line.
- Bend your arms and pull your chest up to touch the bar.
- Extend your arms and return to the starting position without bending your knees or hips.

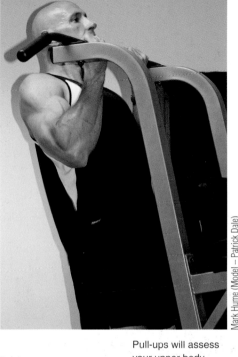

Mark Hume (Model – Patrick Dale)

Pull-ups will assess your upper body pulling strength.

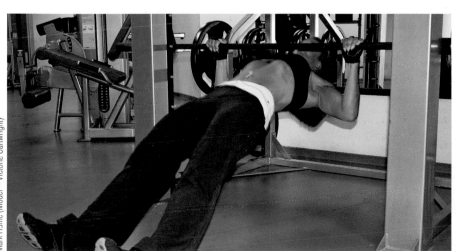

Mark Hume (Model – Victoria Cartwright)

If pull-ups are too challenging, perform body rows instead.

Test three – bent leg sit-ups

Bent leg sit-ups are a bit out of vogue with the mainstream fitness community, who suggest you should work your abs independently of your hip flexors and lower back muscles. This, however, is not the way your core muscles were designed to work! Sit-ups are one of many effective exercises that are often frowned upon but, when included as part of a well-balanced training programme such as this one, are actually quite acceptable. That said, minimize your risk of injury by *never* pulling on the back of your neck and not sitting forwards past vertical.

- Lie on the floor with your legs bent and feet flat – you may need to anchor your feet or have a training partner grasp them for you.
- Place your hands on your temples, across your chest or on your thighs.
- Sit up until your body is upright and perpendicular to the floor. If you are in the first position, your elbows should touch your knees.
- Lower your back down into the starting position and repeat.

Test four – 300 m (330 yard) run

This test will assess your basic running speed, anaerobic fitness and *esprit de corps*. *Esprit de corps*, in the terminology of the Royal Marines, is essentially a 'gut check' to see what you are made of! Run as fast as you can for this test – remember it's a sprint and not a bimble! (Bimble means a slow, aimless walk or run.)

Box burpees ensure that your jumps are the same height each and every rep!

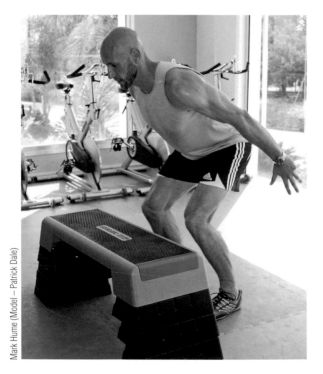

Mark Hume (Model – Patrick Dale)

- Place two marker cones 50 m (55 yards) apart.
- On the command 'Go', sprint out to the first marker cone, touch it with your hand and then sprint back.
- Perform three times to total 300 m (330 yards).

Test five – box burpees

Burpees – the exercise every soldier loves to hate. The burpee combines squats and press-ups into one full-body exercise that will condition all your muscles and drive your heart rate sky-high. The 180-second burpee test is designed to assess your anaerobic fitness and your total-body muscular endurance. To ensure that you don't loaf (take it easy) on any of your reps, this version of burpees is slightly unusual and requires the use of a 30 cm (12 in) high platform.

- Stand around 45 cm (18 in) from your sturdy platform with your feet hip-width apart.
- Squat down and place your hands on the floor just in front of your feet.
- Jump your feet out behind you so you land in the press-up position.
- Perform a single press-up.
- Jump your feet back under you and up to your hands.
- Leap up and forwards to land on the platform.
- Jump back to the floor and repeat – only about 2 minutes and 50 seconds to go!

Troop Phyz Workouts

With the fitness tests now completed, it's time to look to the troop phyz workouts. Some workouts contain exercises that crop up more than once – this is not a misprint. The repeated exercises in this programme are so effective that they simply cannot be improved upon and they form the cornerstone of any good training programme.

Troop Phyz 1 – Spartan Circuit

This is one of my favourite workouts! It ticks lots of fitness component boxes and is easily adaptable according to the equipment you have available. Why the Spartan circuit? It's brutally effective like the Spartan warriors were and it can be performed even when exercise equipment is sparse. Who said the military don't have a sense of humour?

Equipment: timer, skipping rope, exercise mat.
Duration: 30 minutes plus warm-up and cool-down.
Purpose: aerobic conditioning, whole-body muscular endurance.
Method: set your timer for alternating 2 minute and 1 minute intervals and then complete the following circuit twice. This is a continuous circuit, so move from one exercise to the next without taking any rests. If you are not a very proficient skipper, you can substitute jogging or marching on the spot, step-ups, cycling on an exercise bike, running on a treadmill, jumping jacks or any other suitable cardiovascular exercise as an alternative.

- 2 minutes skipping
- 1 minute press-ups
- 2 minutes skipping
- 1 minute squats
- 2 minutes skipping
- 1 minute dorsal raises
- 2 minutes skipping
- 1 minute planks
- 2 minutes skipping
- 1 minute lunges

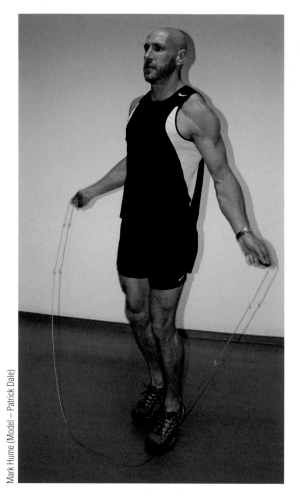

Mark Hume (Model – Patrick Dale)

EXERCISE DESCRIPTIONS
Skipping

Skipping, or jumping rope if you prefer, is a cardiovascular exercise that also improves eye/hand/foot coordination. In this instance, it is being used both as an 'active rest' and for aerobic conditioning. Make sure your rope is the right length for you by standing on the middle with both feet. If the handles reach your armpits then the rope is the right size for you. Too long or too short a rope will increase your likelihood of tripping, which will reduce the effectiveness of this workout.

- Stand with your feet together, your hands at hip-height and the rope behind you.
- Swing it up and over your head.
- Jump over it as it nears your feet – try to only just clear it by jumping no higher than necessary.
- As you get more proficient at jumping rope, try using a heel/toe action or jogging on the spot. It's actually easier and looks much cooler!
- Try to perform your skipping on a forgiving surface to minimize your likelihood of developing any impact-related injuries.

Press-ups

You know how to do these now but, in case you missed it, here is a reminder …

- Bend down and place your hands on the floor, shoulder-width apart. Point your fingers forwards.
- With your arms straight, walk your feet back into the press-up position.
- Check that your heels, hips and shoulders form a straight line.
- Keep your core muscles tight and your neck long – tuck your chin in slightly.
- Bend your elbows and, keeping your arms tucked into your ribs, lower your chest to within 2–3 cm (an inch) of the floor.
- Push back up and return to the starting position.
- If full press-ups are too challenging, bend your legs and place your knees on the floor. This is the three-quarter press-up.
- You can make press-ups more challenging by elevating your feet on a 30–45 cm (12–18 in) high bench.

Squats

Squats are the kings of lower body exercise. Performed with high reps using just your bodyweight they will increase your muscular endurance and lung capacity. Performed with heavy weights and lower reps they will build and strengthen your entire lower body.

- Stand with your feet shoulder-width apart and your hands by your sides.
- Turn your feet out slightly.
- Push your hips back and bend your knees.
- Squat down until your thighs are roughly parallel to the floor.
- Stand back up and repeat.
- Try not to round your lower back at the bottom of the squat as this may lead to injury.

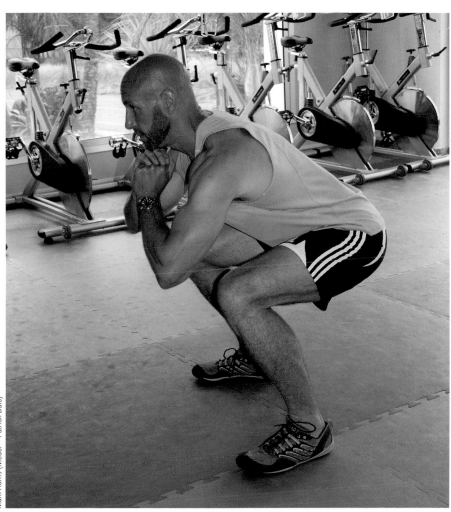

Mark Hume (Model – Patrick Dae)

A shallow squat is a useless squat – do make sure your knees hit 90 degrees!

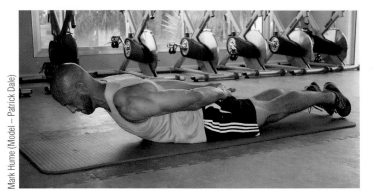

Mark Hume (Model – Patrick Dale)

Dorsal raises

Dorsal raises strengthen and conditioning your lower back and provide a nice balance to any abdominal exercise. Perform this exercise while lying on a mat. Males may also be more comfortable if they place a small cushion under their hips. I'm sure you don't have to ask why ...

Dorsal raises – an effective lower back strengthening exercise

- Lie on your front with your legs extended and held together.
- Clasp your hands behind your back.
- Push your toes into the floor and use your back muscles to lift your head, shoulders and chest around 20-30 cm (8-12 in) off the floor.
- Hold this uppermost position for 1-2 seconds and then return to the starting position.
- You may find you need to place your feet against a wall to help keep your balance.

Planks

Planks are a curious exercise in that, although they do not involve any actual movement, they are still very challenging. Planks will strengthen the anterior or front core muscles.

Planks involve no movement but are nonetheless very challenging and effective.

- Kneel down and place your elbows on the floor, shoulder-width apart.
- Lay your hands flat, with your forearms pointing straight forwards.
- Walk your legs back and extend your legs so that your weight is supported on your arms and feet only.

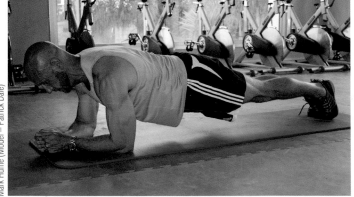

Mark Hume (Model – Patrick Dale)

- Make sure your heels, hips and shoulders are aligned.
- Brace your core muscles and hold this position - do not let your hips drop or your back arch.
- Remember to breathe! Amazingly it's not uncommon for people to forget this vital instruction!

Lunges

Lunges are similar to squats in that they target every muscle in your lower body, but they also challenge your balance and coordination. Lunges simulate the one-legged action of running, which makes them a great addition to your programme. They also make your butt look great in jeans!

- Stand with your feet together and your hands by your sides.
- Take a large step forwards.
- Bend your legs and lower your rear knee to within 2–3 cm (an inch) of the floor.
- Push off your front leg and spring back to the starting position.
- Perform another rep, leading with your opposite leg.
- Continue alternating legs for the duration of your set.

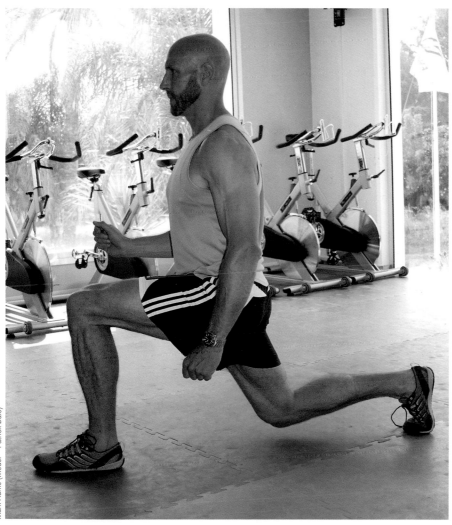

Mark Hume (Model – Patrick Dale)

Lunges – a great butt, leg and balance exercise

Troop Phyz 2 – Para 5/10/15/20 Circuit

Paras love pull-ups – only they call them 'heaves', as do many branches of the military. This all-round muscular endurance workout gets the job done in double-quick time – not unlike the Paras themselves.

Equipment: pull-up bar, exercise mat, timer.
Duration: 20 minutes plus warm-up and cool-down.
Purpose: whole-body muscular endurance.
Method: perform as many laps of the following circuit as you can in 20 minutes. Record the total number of laps completed and aim to beat it next time. Adjust the reps to suit your individual fitness level, e.g. 3/6/9/12 instead of the prescribed 5/10/15/20. You can also make this workout more challenging by increasing the reps to 6/12/18/24 or more.

- 5 pull-ups
- 10 press-ups
- 15 squats
- 20 hill climbers

EXERCISE DESCRIPTIONS
Pull-ups

This is the same exercise that you performed in the fitness tests but, for those of you who missed it, here are your instructions again.

- Grasp an overhead bar with a slightly wider than shoulder-width overhand grip.
- Hang at full stretch with your arms and legs extended – this is called the dead hang position.
- Pull strongly with your arms and lift your chin up and over the bar.
- Slowly lower to the starting position and repeat.

Pull-up option – body rows

If you are unable to perform pull-ups, you can perform body rows instead. This exercise uses similar muscles but the inclined position of your body reduces the effect of gravity somewhat.

- Adjust the bar on a Smith machine or squat rack to hip-height.
- Sit beneath the bar and grasp it with an overhand shoulder-width grip.
- Extend your legs and lift your butt off the floor – your heels, hips and shoulders should form a straight line.
- Bend your arms and pull your chest up to touch the bar.

- Extend your arms and return to the starting position without bending your knees or hips.

Press-ups

You really must have these right by now ...

- Bend down and place your hands on the floor, shoulder-width apart. Point your fingers forwards.
- With your arms straight, walk your feet back into the press-up position.
- Check that your heels, hips and shoulders form a straight line.
- Keep your core muscles tight and your neck long – tuck your chin in slightly.
- Bend your elbows and, keeping your arms tucked into your ribs, lower your chest to within 2–3 cm (an inch) of the floor.
- Push back up and return to the starting position.
- If full press-ups are too challenging, bend your legs and place your knees on the floor. This is the three-quarter press-up.
- You can make press-ups more challenging by elevating your feet on a 30–45 cm (12–18 in) high bench.

Squats

Performed exactly as before ...

- Stand with your feet shoulder-width apart and your hands by your sides.
- Turn your feet out slightly.
- Push your hips back and bend your knees.
- Squat down until your thighs are roughly parallel to the floor.
- Stand back up and repeat.
- Try not to round your lower back at the bottom of the squat as this may lead to injury.

Hill climbers

Hill climbers, sometimes called single-leg squat thrusts, are an excellent exercise for driving your heart rate up and conditioning your legs. Go for a big range of movement to get the most from this effective manoeuvre.

- Adopt the press-up position with your arms extended and your heels, hips and shoulders aligned.

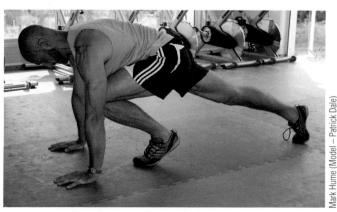

Hill climbers – pump your legs as fast as you can!

Mark Hume (Model – Patrick Dale)

- Bend one leg and draw your knee towards your chest – this is your starting position.
- Jump your forward leg back while simultaneously jumping your rear leg forwards.
- Repeat the movement so you are back in your starting position – this constitutes 1 rep.
- Continue for the prescribed number of reps but remember to count the reps on one leg only or you'll end up doing half as many as you should!

Troop Phyz 3 – Deck of Cards Workout

Decks of cards and dice are one of the ways that unpleasant jobs are allocated in the armed forces. Junior ranks often have to cut the cards or roll the dice to see who is on coffee-making duty or, worse still, kitchen duty. The thrill of anticipation is unavoidable as you turn over a card to reveal that you won't be the poor squaddie scrubbing pots all evening. This workout is a homage to this particular military tradition.

Equipment: deck of playing cards, exercise mat, stopwatch.
Duration: against the clock.
Purpose: whole-body muscular endurance and aerobic conditioning.
Method: take your deck of cards and give them a good shuffle. Place the pack face down. Turn the top card face up and perform the exercise allocated for the value of the card, e.g. six of hearts = 6 squats, queen of clubs = 12 press-ups. Work through the entire pack as fast as possible but only move on to the next card when you have completed all of the reps of your current card. If you get a run of high cards or same-colour cards ... bad luck!
Red cards = squats
Black cards = press-ups (full, or on knees, as appropriate)
Jokers = 20 burpees
Values: 1 to 10 = 1 to 10 reps, picture cards (jacks, kings, queens) = 12 reps

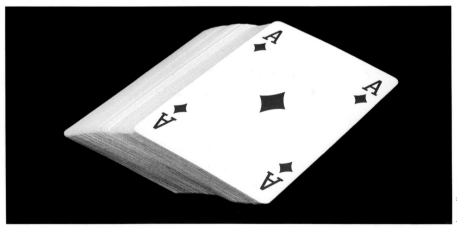

A deck of playing cards can be used as the basis for a workout.

dreamstime.com

Military Fitness

EXERCISE DESCRIPTIONS
Squats
Practice makes perfect, or so they say, so you should be scoring 10 out of 10 for squats by now ...

- Stand with your feet shoulder-width apart and your hands by your sides.
- Turn your feet out slightly.
- Push your hips back and bend your knees.
- Squat down until your thighs are roughly parallel to the floor.
- Stand back up and repeat.
- Try not to round your lower back at the bottom of the squat as this may lead to injury.

Press-ups
You'll be performing a lot of repetitions of press-ups in this workout so don't let your technique suffer and run the risk of an otherwise avoidable injury or, worse still, an inefficient workout!

- Bend down and place your hands on the floor, shoulder-width apart. Point your fingers forwards.
- With your arms straight, walk your feet back into the press-up position.
- Check that your heels, hips and shoulders form a straight line.
- Keep your core muscles tight and your neck long – tuck your chin in slightly.
- Bend your elbows and, keeping your arms tucked into your ribs, lower your chest to within 2-3 cm (an inch) of the floor.
- Push back up and return to the starting position.
- If full press-ups are too challenging, bend your legs and place your knees on the floor. This is the three-quarter press-up.
- You can make press-ups more challenging by elevating your feet on a 30-45 cm (12-18 in) high bench.

Burpees
You only have to perform two sets of burpees in this entire workout so make each rep count by doing them with the best technique you can muster. Make your old PTI proud:

- Squat down and place your hands on the floor just in front of your feet.
- Jump your feet out behind you so you land in the press-up position.
- Perform a single press-up.
- Jump your feet back under you and up to your hands.
- Leap up into the air as high as you can.

- On landing, immediately drop into another rep.
- Try not to land like a baby elephant when doing this exercise – stay on your toes and, although you are jumping as high as you can, make sure you land as lightly as possible.

Troop Phyz Workout 4 – Samurai Tabata Circuit

Fearsome warriors, the Japanese Samurai would only re-sheathe their swords once they had drawn blood and would commit ritual suicide if ordered to do so, or if they felt their honour had been shamed. Thankfully, this workout is not going to result in any blood being spilt but it will certainly test your mettle.

Equipment: exercise mat, skipping rope, timer.
Duration: 30 minutes plus warm-up and cool-down.
Purpose: whole-body muscular endurance, anaerobic conditioning.
Method: Tabata training uses 20-second work periods alternated with 10-second rests repeated for 10 sets and totalling 5 minutes. For this workout you will be performing five Tabata exercises, one after another with a 1-minute rest between exercises. Try to perform as many reps as you can for each exercise. Make a note of your rep totals per exercise and try to beat that score next time you perform this workout.

The five exercises are:

1. **Burpees** (10 sets of 20 seconds work, 10 seconds recovery)
   1 minute rest
2. **Crunches** (10 sets of 20 seconds work, 10 seconds recovery)
   1 minute rest
3. **Skipping** – knee lift sprint (10 sets of 20 seconds work, 10 seconds recovery)
   1 minute rest
4. **Thrusters** (10 sets of 20 seconds work, 10 seconds recovery)
   1 minute rest
5. **Kettlebell/dumbbell swings** (10 sets of 20 seconds work, 10 seconds recovery)

EXERCISE DESCRIPTIONS
Burpees

You will be performing a higher volume of burpees in this workout separated by only short rests. Don't forget to focus on good exercise technique to get the most from your training session and avoid any unnecessary injuries, aches and pains.

- Squat down and place your hands on the floor just in front of your feet.
- Jump your feet out behind you so you land in the press-up position.

- Perform a single press-up.
- Jump your feet back under you and up to your hands.
- Leap up into the air as high as you can.
- On landing, immediately drop into another rep.
- Try not to land like a baby elephant when doing this exercise – stay on your toes and, although you are jumping as high as you can, make sure you land as lightly as possible.

Crunches

Crunches, like sit-ups, come in for a bit of stick from many trainers in the fitness industry. The truth is that they are an effective anterior core exercise that will strengthen and condition your rectus abdominis or abs for short. The secret to successful crunch performance is to do them slowly and really *squeeze* your abs as though you are trying to wring them dry! Remember, no pulling on your neck.

- Lie on your back with your legs bent and feet flat on the floor.
- Place your hands on your temples, across your chest or on your thighs.
- Exhale and raise your head, shoulders and upper back off the floor.
- *Squeeze* for two to five seconds!
- Return to the starting position and repeat.
- You can also perform this exercise with your feet elevated and your knees and hips flexed to 90 degrees.

Crunch and squeeze your abs as hard as you can for best six-pack-building results!

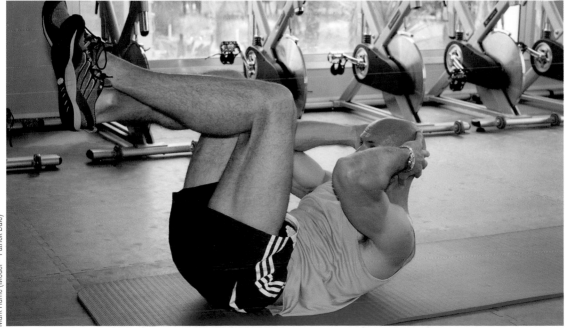

Mark Hume (Model – Patrick Dale)

Skipping – knee lift sprint

The last time you did this exercise you performed it at a slow to moderate pace as an aerobic conditioner and recovery opportunity. This time you are going to perform it as an anaerobic interval.

- Begin skipping normally and then make a transition to jogging on the spot.
- Keep your body upright and lift your knees so that your thighs are parallel to the floor.
- Pump your legs as fast as you can as you spin your rope.
- This exercise is more challenging – especially if you are new to skipping. Persevere, practise skipping whenever you get the chance and you'll soon be skipping like a pro.

Thrusters

Combining squats and shoulder presses, thrusters provide real 'bang for your buck'.

Thrusters combine a squat with a shoulder press to target your legs, arms and midsection. They will also challenge your cardiovascular system. You can perform this exercise using dumbbells, a barbell, a medicine ball, kettlebell or sandbag – even a large rock!

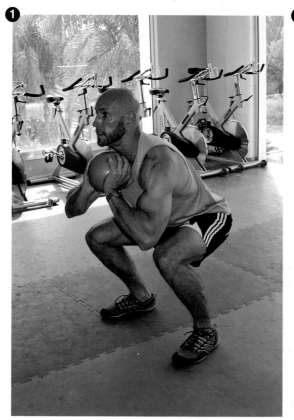

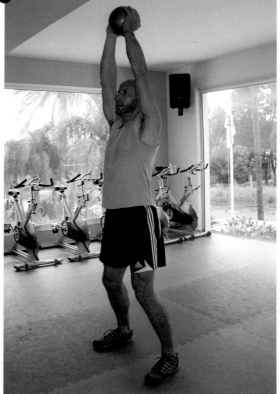

Mark Hume (Model – Patrick Dale)

- Stand with your feet shoulder-width apart with your chosen weight in your hands.
- Raise the weight to chest level so it is resting in your upturned palms and your elbows are down by your chest.
- Squat down so that your thighs are parallel to the floor.
- Drive up out of the squat and use the momentum from your legs to push the weight overhead to arms' length.
- Lower the weight back to your chest and then descend into another squat.

Kettlebell/dumbbell swings

The final exercise in this workout is the kettlebell swing. Don't worry if you don't have access to a kettlebell though – you can perform this exercise with a dumbbell or a medicine ball in a strong bag as necessary. Kettlebell swings strengthen your hips, hamstrings and lower back and are one of the best butt exercises you can do.

- Stand with your feet shoulder-width apart and your weight held in front of your thighs.
- Bend your knees slightly and then hinge forwards from your hips.
- Lower the weight between your knees.
- Drive your hips forwards and swing the weight at arms' length up to between chest and head height. The hip drive in this exercise is not dissimilar to the take-off for a standing long jump. Keep this in your mind to maximize the effectiveness of this exercise.
- Do not allow your lower back to round at any point during this exercise.

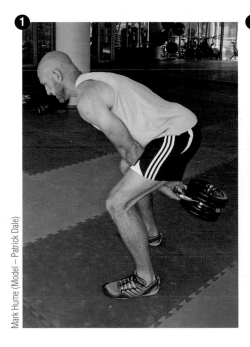

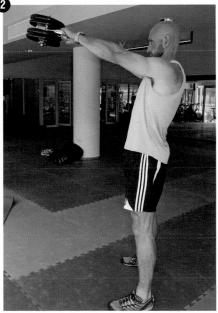

Drive your hips into your swings for best effect!

Troop Phyz 5 – Parade Square Corners

Drill instructors will be turning in their graves if you dare violate their parade squares to perform PT! To the DL or Drill Leader, the parade square is sacred ground on which you must march with the correct military bearing and never just walk. Drill – marching in formation – is a regular part of armed forces life that teaches teamwork and group cohesion. Maybe you can simulate this by performing this workout with a group of like-minded training buddies? Adjust the reps to suit your individual fitness level.

Equipment: soccer pitch or similar, timer.
Duration: 20 minutes plus warm-up and cool-down.
Purpose: aerobic conditioning, whole-body muscular endurance.
Method: complete as many laps as possible of the following circuit – *perform 25 reps of each 'corner' exercise.*

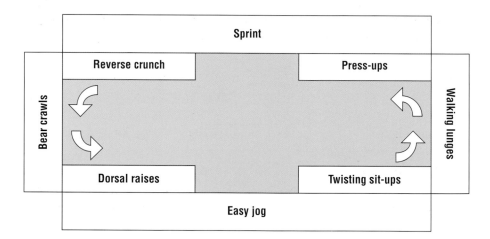

EXERCISE DESCRIPTIONS
Press-ups

Surely by now you must be doing these pretty well? Be careful where you put your hands if you are performing this workout in a doggy-frequented park ...

- Bend down and place your hands on the floor, shoulder-width apart. Point your fingers forwards.
- With your arms straight, walk your feet back into the press-up position.
- Check that your heels, hips and shoulders form a straight line.
- Keep your core muscles tight and your neck long – tuck your chin in slightly.
- Bend your elbows and, keeping your arms tucked into your ribs, lower your chest to within 2–3 cm (an inch) of the floor.
- Push back up and return to the starting position.

- If full press-ups are too challenging, bend your legs and place your knees on the floor. This is the three-quarter press-up.
- You can make press-ups more challenging by elevating your feet on a 30–45 cm (12-18 in) high bench.

Sprints

Sprints will condition your legs and raise your heart rate as well as making the next exercise much more demanding.

- Pump your arms and drive hard with your legs to cover the ground as fast as possible.
- Lean forwards slightly and try to stay up on your toes.

Reverse crunches

While there is no such thing as your lower abdominals, you can initiate an abdominal contraction by raising your hips instead of raising your shoulders. Your legs are pretty heavy so don't be surprised if you find this exercise challenging.

- Lie on your back with your knees and hips flexed to 90 degrees.
- Rest your arms on the floor, slightly away from your sides, with your palms facing up.
- Without using your arms (hence the arm and hand position) curl your hips up and lift your butt off the floor.
- Hold this position for 1–2 seconds and then return to the starting position.
- This movement is relatively small – any big movements will result in hip flexion rather than spine flexion. Spine flexion works your core muscles; hip flexion does not.

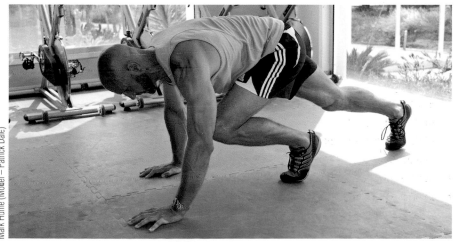

Mark Hume (Model – Patrick Dale)

Bear crawls – an effective total-body exercise

Bear crawls

This exercise will develop your muscular endurance, leg and core strength. Military types spend a fair amount of their basic training crawling – usually on their bellies through water-filled trenches using a technique called the leopard crawl. The bear crawl is slightly different in that you don't have to drag your belly through the mud. Different, but not easier ...

- Bend down and adopt the press-up position.
- Lift your hips, bend your knees and look forwards.
- Using an opposite arm and leg movement, crawl forwards as fast as you can.

Dorsal raises

You've done them before but they are such an effective lower back exercise that they are worth repeating. Check the floor for debris before lying face down.

- Lie on your front with your legs extended and held together.
- Clasp your hands behind your back.
- Push your toes into the floor and use your back muscles to lift your head, shoulders and chest around 20-30 cm (8-12 in) off the floor.
- Hold this uppermost position for 1-2 seconds and then return to the starting position.
- You may find you need to hold your feet in place to help keep your balance.

Easy jog

Adopt the 'commando shuffle' and use this exercise as an active recovery. The slower you run, the longer your rest – but also the longer the workout will last!

- Jog slowly to the next corner.
- Stay low to the ground.
- Use short strides.
- Keep your upper body relaxed.
- Try to get your breathing under control.

Twisting sit-ups

Yet another slightly frowned-upon exercise that is actually a very effective midsection conditioning exercise. Avoid sitting up past vertical and only twist as far as is comfortable to minimize your risk of discomfort or injury.

- Lie on the ground with your legs bent and feet flat on the floor.
- Place your hands next to your temples, with your elbows spread wide.
- Sit up and twist your left elbow towards your right knee.

- Return to the starting position and then sit up but turn your right elbow to your left knee.
- Continue alternating sides for the duration of your set.

Walking lunges

Walking lunges, like regular lunges, are an effective lower body exercise. The main advantage of walking lunges is the emphasis they place on the muscles at the back of your thigh and hip - specifically your glutes and hamstrings. These muscles are essential in all walking and running activities and need to be kept strong.

- Stand with your feet together and your hands by your sides.
- Take a large step forwards, bend your legs and lower your rear knee to within 2–3 cm (an inch) of the floor.
- Stand up and step through straight into another rep.
- Continue lunging until you have covered the prescribed distance.

Troop Phyz Workout 6 – *Per Mare, Per Terram*

The Royal Marine Commandos are the UK's 'go anywhere, do anything' amphibious troops who are just as at home on skis as they are storming a beach or hacking through jungles. The ability of the Marines to work in just about any environment is one of the reasons they are considered amongst the world's most elite military units. This workout is a homage to the Royal Marines' motto '*Per mare, per terram*' which means 'By sea, by land'.

Equipment: rowing machine, exercise bike, treadmill, stopwatch.
Duration: against the clock.
Purpose: aerobic conditioning.
Method: this workout is a straight race against yourself and the clock. Perform each discipline as fast as possible, including the transitions between exercises - the time starts when you begin rowing and ends when you finish running. Although speed is of the essence, make sure you don't set off so fast that you fail to finish. Record your time and try to beat it when you repeat this workout.

1. Row 2,000 m (2,200 yards)
2. Cycle 5,000 m (5,500 yards)
3. Run 2,000 m (2,200 yards)

EXERCISE DESCRIPTIONS

Row 2,000 m (2,200 yards)

Rowing is an effective all-over cardiovascular exercise. As rowing machines vary from model to model you should view these instructions as technique rather than operational guidelines.

- Set the rowing computer to 2,000 m.
- Fix your feet to the foot plates so that the strap is across the broadest part of your feet.
- Grasp the handle with an overhand grip.
- Bend your knees, extend your arms and sit up tall – this is your starting position.
- Drive hard with your legs and, as the handle crosses your knees, begin to pull with your arms.
- Continue pulling until the handle touches your abdomen.
- Extend your arms, bend your legs and slide forwards to return to the starting position.
- Do not allow your lower back to round as this can lead to injury.

Drive with your legs and then pull with your arms, or your arms will tire first!

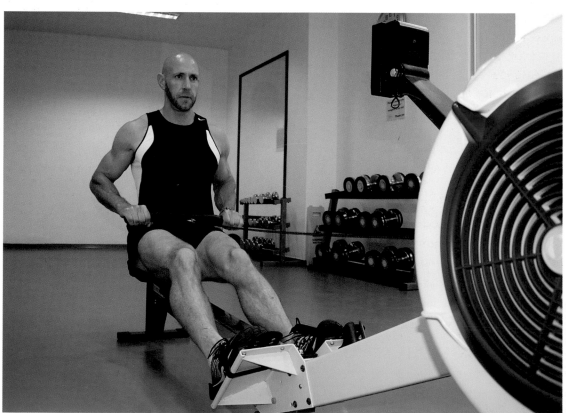

Mark Hume (Model – Patrick Dale)

Cycle 5,000 m (5,500 yards)

This simple cardiovascular exercise can all go horribly wrong if you don't set up your bike correctly! Professional cyclists spend weeks in wind tunnels making sure they are properly positioned on the bike. Make sure you spend a few seconds to ensure that you are set up properly too! Do this prior to starting the workout to save transition time.

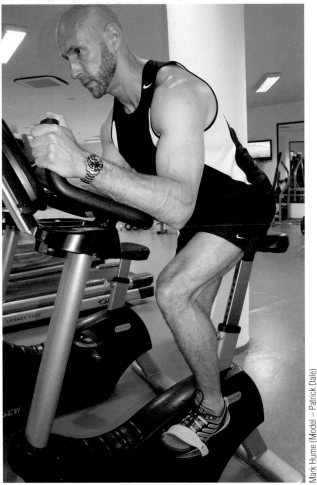

- Stand next to the bike and adjust the seat so that it is level with your hip.
- Sit on the bike and place your feet in the pedal straps. The balls of your feet should be directly aligned with the pivot point of the pedal.
- Push one leg all the way down – you should have a slight bend in your knee and should not need to rock over.
- Repeat this process with the other leg in case you have a leg length discrepancy.
- Place your hands on the handlebars, set the distance on the bike computer and begin pedalling.
- Try to keep your upper body relaxed and avoid rocking from side to side – this is uneconomical and can make cycling uncomfortable.

Mark Hume (Model – Patrick Dale)

No resting during the bike ride – work as hard as you can.

Run 2,000 m (2,200 yards)

Your legs may be feeling decidedly jelly-like now and the only way you will get them feeling even halfway normal is to set off on your run at a good, fast pace. Starting off slowly merely delays the recovery of your leg muscles. As each treadmill operates differently, use these instructions as a guide to running technique.

- Stand on the centre of the belt near the front.
- Start the treadmill and quickly progress from a walk to a jog to a run.
- Focus on a light footfall while using a heel-toe action and keeping your upper body relaxed.
- Stay fairly close to the front of the treadmill so you can hit the emergency stop button if you get into trouble.

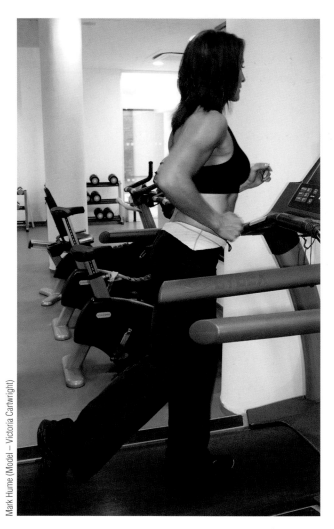

Mark Hume (Model – Victoria Cartwright)

Troop Phyz Workout 7 – Dirty Dozen

The Dirty Dozen were a fictional commando unit made up from military convicts given a last-chance offer to fight the Germans or face the firing squad. These tough, ruthless men went on to cause immeasurable damage to the German military machine and, almost to a man, died heroes. The Dirty Dozen may be fictional but this workout will push you like a real-life angry sergeant-major.

Equipment: rowing machine, exercise mat, pull-up bar, step box, 20 kg (44 lb) dumbbell or kettlebell, treadmill, skipping rope, 15 kg (33 lb) dumbbells, stopwatch.
Duration: against the clock.
Purpose: whole-body muscular endurance, anaerobic conditioning.
Method: storm through this list of exercises as fast as possible. Rest when necessary, but the clock keeps on ticking so no dilly-dallying! Adjust the weights and reps to suit your individual fitness level. Record the time it takes you to complete this workout and try to beat it when you repeat it in a few weeks' time.

The faster you run, the sooner your legs will feel better!

1. Row 500 m (550 yards)
2. Burpees x 12
3. Pull-ups x 12
4. Plyometric press-ups x 12
5. 60 cm (24 in) box jumps x 24
6. Kettlebell/dumbbell swings @ 20 kg (44 lb) x 24
7. Run 400 m (440 yards) @ 5% incline
8. Bent leg sit-ups x 24
9. Press-ups x 24
10. Double-unders x 24
11. Dumbbell curl and press @ 15 kg (33 lb) x 12
12. Kneeling squat jumps x 24

EXERCISE DESCRIPTIONS

Row

You rowed 2,000 m (2,200 yards) in the previous workout but this time, instead of a long grind, you'll be completing a 500 m (550 yard) all-out sprint!

- Set the rowing computer to 500 m.
- Fix your feet to the foot plates so that the strap is across the broadest part of your feet.
- Grasp the handle with an overhand grip.
- Bend your knees, extend your arms and sit up tall – this is your starting position.
- Drive hard with your legs and, as the handle crosses your knees, begin to pull with your arms.
- Continue pulling until the handle touches your abdomen.
- Extend your arms, bend your legs and slide forwards to return to the starting position.
- Do not allow your lower back to round as this can lead to injury.

Burpees

Do you love them or hate them? Either way, burpees are one of the ultimate all-round conditioning exercises.

- Squat down and place your hands on the floor just in front of your feet.
- Jump your feet out behind you so you land in the press-up position.
- Perform a single press-up.
- Jump your feet back under you and up to your hands.
- Leap up into the air as high as you can.
- On landing, immediately drop into another rep.
- Try not to land like a baby elephant when doing this exercise – stay on your toes and, although you are jumping as high as you can, make sure you land as lightly as possible.

Pull-ups

Build your arms and back with this effective upper body exercise. This is the same exercise that you performed in the fitness tests but, for those of you who missed it, here are your instructions again:

- Grasp an overhead bar with a slightly wider than shoulder-width overhand grip.
- Hang at full stretch with your arms and legs extended – this is called the dead hang position.
- Pull strongly with your arms and lift your chin up and over the bar.
- Slowly lower to the starting position and repeat.

Option – body rows

If you are unable to perform pull-ups, you can do body rows instead. This exercise uses similar muscles but the inclined position of your body reduces the effect of gravity somewhat.

- Adjust the bar on a Smith machine or squat rack to hip-height.
- Sit beneath the bar and grasp it with an overhand shoulder-width grip.
- Extend your legs and lift your butt off the floor – your heels, hips and shoulders should form a straight line.
- Bend your arms and pull your chest up to touch the bar.
- Extend your arms and return to the starting position without bending your knees or hips.

Plyometric press-ups

Plyometric or clap press-ups take press-ups to a whole new level – literally! This more advanced variation of the exercise you know and love will develop muscle power rather than endurance (as is the case with regular press-ups).

- Adopt the regular press-up position with your hands shoulder-width apart and your weight supported on your hands and toes only. Keep your core muscles braced throughout.
- Bend your arms and lower your chest to within 2–3 cm (an inch) of the floor and keep your elbows tucked into your ribs.
- Extend your arms explosively and drive your upper body off, up and away from the floor.
- Clap your hands while you are in mid-air.
- On landing, bend your arms and descend immediately into another rep.

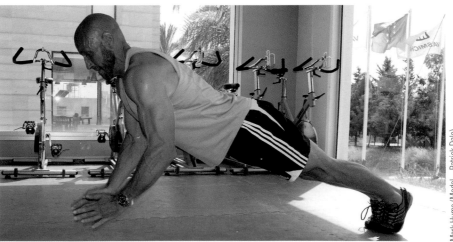

Plyo press-ups – get some air!

Mark Hume (Model – Patrick Dale)

60 cm (24 in) box jumps

Box jumps develop leg power in the same way that plyometric press-ups develop arm power. This effective exercise will increase your explosive strength, which will translate to faster running and higher jumping ability. Adjust the height of your box according to your current jumping ability.

- Stand 45 cm (18 in) from your box.
- Bend your knees and descend into a quarter-depth squat position.
- Extend your arms behind you.
- Swing your arms dynamically forwards and jump forwards and upwards on to your box.
- Aim to land with both feet squarely on the box-top.
- Step down and repeat.
- Alternate the leg you use to step down to ensure you don't end up with one leg better developed than the other!

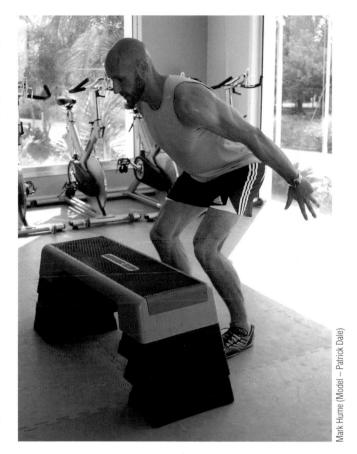

Mark Hume (Model – Patrick Dale)

Jump up and then step back down to save your knees.

Kettlebell/dumbbell swings

This champion hip and butt exercise is back – remember you can perform it using a single dumbbell or any other appropriate weight.

- Stand with your feet shoulder-width apart and your weight held in front of your thighs.
- Bend your knees slightly and then hinge forwards from your hips.
- Lower the weight between your knees.
- Drive your hips forwards and swing the weight at arms' length up to between chest and head height. The hip drive in this exercise is not dissimilar to the take-off for a standing long jump. Keep this in your mind to maximize the effectiveness of this exercise.
- Do not allow your lower back to round at any point during this exercise.
- Adjust the weight according to your personal fitness level.

Run 400 m (440 yards) at 5% incline

A fairly self-explanatory exercise – simply run fast uphill. Sounds easier than it actually is!

- Stand on the centre of the belt near the front.
- Start the treadmill and quickly progress from a walk to a jog to a run as you simultaneously increase the incline.
- Focus on a light footfall, using a heel-toe action and keeping your upper body relaxed.
- Stay fairly close to the front of the treadmill so you can hit the emergency stop button if you get into trouble.
- Treat this as a sprint – although, in reality, this is more likely to become a run for survival!

Bent leg sit-ups

You know how to do these now, but performing this exercise while severely out of breath adds a whole new dimension. Try to time your panting with your reps and don't be surprised if you have to break your set down into smaller groups of reps because of residual fatigue caused by the run. Remember, regardless of how tired you are, no pulling on your neck.

- Lie on the floor with your legs and feet flat – you may need to anchor your feet or have a training partner grasp them for you.
- Place your hands on your temples, across your chest or on your thighs.
- Sit up until your body is upright and perpendicular to the floor. If you are in the first position, your elbows should touch your knees.
- Lower back down into the starting position and repeat.

Press-ups

Like the sit-ups before, performing press-ups when out of breath can really add to the challenge. Focus on your technique and grind out the reps. There's nothing wrong with resting on your knees for a second or two but don't dilly-dally or the PTI will have your guts for garters for loafing.

- Bend down and place your hands on the floor, shoulder-width apart. Point your fingers forwards.
- With your arms straight, walk your feet back into the press-up position.
- Check that your heels, hips and shoulders form a straight line.
- Keep your core muscles tight and your neck long – tuck your chin in slightly.
- Bend your elbows and, keeping your arms tucked into your ribs, lower your chest to within 2-3 cm (an inch) of the floor.

- Push back up and return to the starting position.
- If full press-ups are too challenging, bend your legs and place your knees on the floor. This is the three-quarter press-up.
- You can make press-ups more challenging by elevating your feet on a 30–45 cm (12–18 in) high bench.

Double-unders

By now you should be a reasonably proficient skipper. While you might not be floating like a butterfly and stinging like a bee, you should at least be able to skip for a few minutes without falling over your own feet. Double-unders will push your skipping ability up a level and will do the same thing to your heart rate and fitness levels.

- Skip normally to get the rope moving – these do not count but are merely the lead-in to the main exercise.
- Increase the speed of your rope turns and perform two rope turns per jump.
- Try not to jump too high – double-unders are achieved more with increased rope speed than with elevated jumping height.
- Avoid landing like a newbie Para on his first parachute jump – stay on your toes and stay light on your feet.

Dumbbell curl and press

Biceps, triceps and shoulders are the muscles doing most of the work in this exercise. Your core muscles are also called into play to support your spine. Try not to

Dumbbell curl and press – combining three exercises into one makes the most of your exercise time!

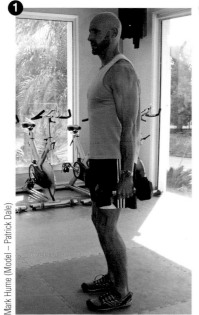
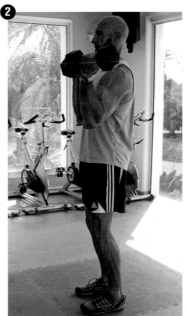
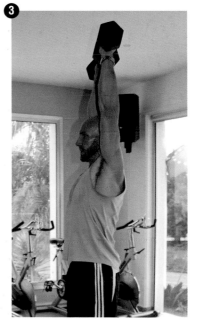

Mark Hume (Model – Patrick Dale)

swing and sway to lift the weights but, instead, concentrate on using arms and shoulders to do the work. Likewise, do not try to 'jerk' the weight above your head like a weightlifter. This isn't the Olympic final you know!

- Grasp a dumbbell in each hand and then stand with your feet hip-width apart and your hands by your sides.
- Bend your knees slightly and brace your core muscles.
- Flex your arms and raise the weights up to shoulder level.

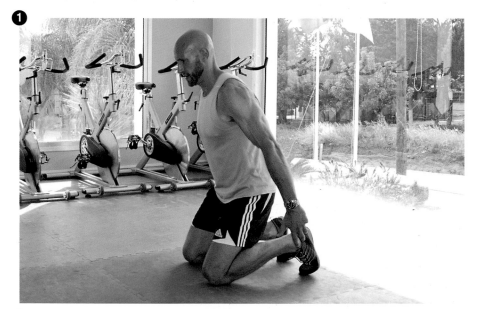

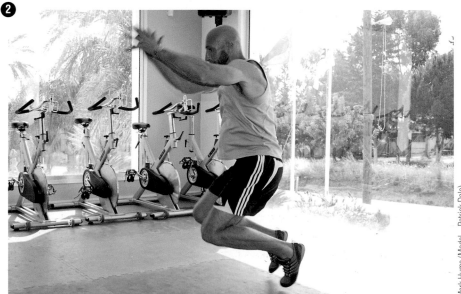

Kneeling squat jumps will challenge your heart and lungs!

- Press the weights above your head to arms' length.
- Bend your arms and lower the dumbbells back to your shoulders.
- Lower the weights all the way down to the starting position.
- Repeat for the prescribed number of reps.
- Adjust the weight of the dumbbells to suit your individual fitness level.

Kneeling squat jumps

This equipment-free lower body exercise is tough on your quads and glutes and will also raise your heart rate. Try to establish a brisk rhythm and stick with it – remember this *is* the last exercise in this workout!

- Kneel down on an exercise mat with your butt close to your heels.
- Thrust your arms forwards and jump from your knees into a low squat position.
- Keeping your legs bent and your butt low, step back and place one knee and then the other on the floor and return to the starting position.
- Immediately perform another rep and continue for the duration of your set.
- Try alternating your leading leg when making the transition from the squat back to the starting position.

Troop Phyz 8 – Bootneck Shuffle

The term 'bootneck' is often used to described the men of the Royal Marines. This harks back to when the Marines were employed upon ships as on-board security and as sharp shooters and wore uniforms with high, stiff leather collars. The bootneck shuffle is a reference to the running gait that Marine recruits (called 'nods' for their ability to fall asleep at any opportunity) adopt early on in their training. The bootneck shuffle is a very economical running style born out of necessity. The large amount of kit carried by the Marines while on patrol means that a more 'bouncy' traditional running style is impossible, so the Marines 'shuffle' along, using a fast foot strike and staying low to the ground. Although you won't need to adopt the bootneck shuffle for this workout, the chances are that, in the days following, your sore glutes, quads and hamstrings will make it a necessity!

Equipment: 400 m (440 yard) running track, stopwatch.
Duration: against the clock.
Purpose: lower body and upper body muscular endurance, mental toughness.
Method: alternate between 20 walking lunges and 20 press-ups and work your way around the circumference of the running track. Rest when necessary, but the clock keeps ticking so don't dawdle! Make sure you perform the press-ups exactly where the lunges finish and vice versa. Make a note of your time and try to beat it when you repeat this workout. If you don't have access to a running track, measure out 400 m (440 yards) on a playing field or similar.

EXERCISE DESCRIPTIONS
Walking lunges

You'll be doing a lot of walking lunges during this workout, so make sure your technique is solid. This is especially important as you begin to fatigue. Tired legs sometimes have a mind of their own, so pay extra attention to the tracking of your knees and position of your torso - no leaning forwards and no pushing off your legs with your arms!

- Stand with your feet together and your hands by your sides.
- Take a large step forwards, bend your legs and lower your rear knee to within 2–3 cm (an inch) of the floor.
- Stand up and step through straight into another rep.
- Continue lunging until you have covered the prescribed distance.

Press-ups

It's safe to say you know how to do a perfect press-up now. Like the lunges, you'll be doing a lot of them in this workout so focus on good exercise performance to minimize injury potential while increasing fitness benefits.

- Bend down and place your hands on the floor, shoulder-width apart. Point your fingers forwards.
- With your arms straight, walk your feet back into the press-up position.
- Check that your heels, hips and shoulders form a straight line.
- Keep your core muscles tight and your neck long - tuck your chin in slightly.
- Bend your elbows and, keeping your arms tucked into your ribs, lower your chest to within 2–3 cm (an inch) of the floor.
- Push back up and return to the starting position.
- If full press-ups are too challenging, bend your legs and place your knees on the floor. This is the three-quarter press-up.

Troop Phyz 9 – Five Centurions

The Five Centurions is dedicated to the Roman legions. One of the first citizen armies manned entirely by professional soldiers, the fitness, strength, discipline and tactics of the Roman legions saw them conquer much of the known world. Centurions had command of 100 men and led their troops by unwavering example - the alternative was death by crucifixion! This simple but effective circuit combines five challenging exercises performed for five 100-rep laps, hence the title. Perform this workout against the clock but don't be surprised if you need to take short breaks between exercises (or even between reps) as this workout is designed to test your mettle. Strive to beat your time on subsequent attempts at this workout.

Equipment: skipping rope, medicine ball, kettlebell/dumbbell, barbell/resistance band and stopwatch.

Duration: against the clock.

Purpose: whole-body muscular endurance, strength, anaerobic fitness.

Method: storm through 5 laps of the following circuit to total 500 reps. Take breaks as necessary but remember this is a race against the clock.

5 laps as fast as possible

20 burpees

20 medicine ball slams

20 double-unders

20 kettlebell swings

20 high pulls

EXERCISE DESCRIPTIONS

Burpees

Burpees will quickly crank up your heart rate and keep it elevated for the duration of this circuit. Focus on good technique, especially as you begin to fatigue, to minimize your risk of injury and maximize the benefits of this grade-A total-body conditioner.

- Squat down and place your hands on the floor just in front of your feet.
- Jump your feet out behind you so you land in the press-up position.
- Perform a single press-up.
- Jump your feet back under you and up to your hands.
- Leap up into the air as high as you can.
- On landing, immediately drop into another rep.
- Try not to land like a baby elephant when doing this exercise – stay on your toes and, although you are jumping as high as you can, make sure you land as lightly as possible.

Medicine ball slams

This is a fun exercise that targets all the muscles on the front of your body. Use a non-gel-filled ball for slams as gel-filled balls have a tendency to burst. If you don't have a medicine ball and are happy to train outside, you can substitute hammer swings (detailed in Chapter 6) or use a sandbag.

- Hold your medicine ball and stand with your feet shoulder-width apart.
- Raise the ball above your head and stretch up on your tiptoes.
- Drop on to your heels and, keeping your arms straight, hurl the medicine ball down at a point around 60 cm (24 in) in front of your feet.

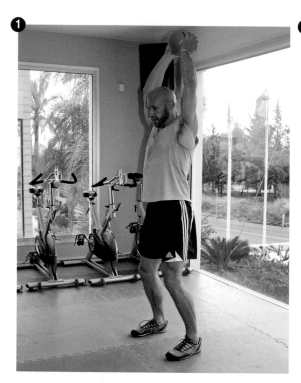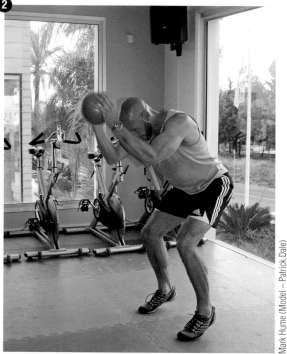

Mark Hume (Model – Patrick Dale)

Throw it like you want to break it!

- Catch the ball as it rebounds off the floor and repeat.
- Try to use your entire body to hurl the ball and not just your arms – imagine your body is the bow and the ball is the arrow.

Double-unders

Double unders will test your skipping ability to the max but, if the truth be told, if you can do these in the middle of a crowded gym you'll look very cool indeed!

- Skip normally to get the rope moving – these do not count but are merely the lead-in to the main exercise.
- Increase the speed of your rope turns and perform two rope turns per jump.
- Try not to jump too high – double-unders are achieved more with increased rope speed than with jumping height.
- Avoid landing like a newbie Para on his first parachute jump – stay on your toes and stay light on your feet.

Kettlebell swings

Kettlebell swings will kick your heart rate up another notch while targeting your all-important glutes, hamstrings and lower back muscles. Focus on a powerful hip thrust rather than trying to 'muscle' the weight up using your arms. Remember, if you don't have a kettlebell, you can use a single dumbbell instead.

- Stand with your feet shoulder-width apart and your weight held in front of your thighs.
- Bend your knees slightly and then hinge forwards from your hips.
- Lower the weight between your knees.
- Drive your hips forwards and swing the weight at arms' length up to between chest and head height. The hip drive in this exercise is not dissimilar to the take-off for a standing long jump. Keep this in your mind to maximize the effectiveness of this exercise.
- Do not allow your lower back to round at any point during this exercise.

High pulls

High pulls can be performed using a barbell, a kettlebell or a resistance band. Whichever you use, choose a light to moderate weight for this exercise as it's very demanding and uses just about every muscle in your lower body. The high pull uses your quads a little more than the kettlebell swings and also requires a strong arm pull, which targets your biceps.

Use your legs as much as possible when performing the high pull.

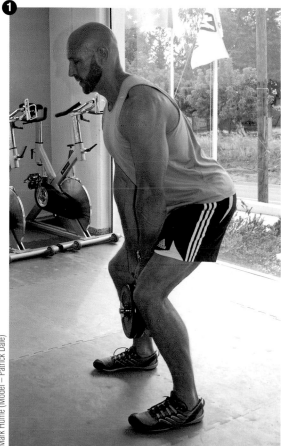

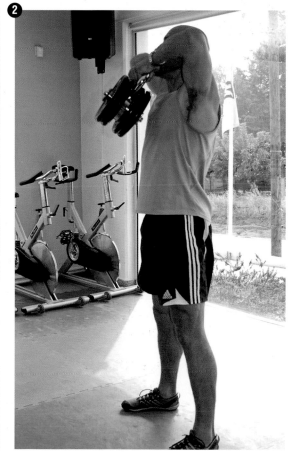

- Stand with your feet shoulder-width apart and the weight held in front of your thighs.
- Push your hips back, bend your legs and lower the weight between your knees.
- Extend your legs and hips explosively and simultaneously pull your hands up and under your chin.
- Lower the weight back to the front of your thighs, bend your knees and repeat.
- Like rowing, try to use your stronger leg muscles as much as possible and use your arms to maintain the momentum generated by the powerful lower body thrust.

Troop Phyz 10 – 5BX

The military loves acronyms. It's like a secret code to ensure that civilians have no idea what you are talking about. You can normally pick out soldiers from civvies simply by listening to the way they speak to each other. It sounds like English and yet they aren't making any sense! Common acronyms include BFT - Basic Fitness Test, ATH - Above The Horizon, ROE - Rules Of Engagement, PFC - Private, First-Class and now 5BX!

Equipment: exercise mat, skipping rope, timer.
Duration: 25 minutes plus warm-up and cool-down.
Purpose: muscular endurance, anaerobic conditioning.
Method: 5BX stands for 5 Basic Exercises and is a common workout in Royal Marine-style circuit training. Perform each of the exercises below for 5 sets using 30/30 intervals, i.e. work for 30 seconds, rest for 30 seconds to a total of 5 minutes per exercise. Move from one exercise to the next without any rest. Perform as many reps as you can during each interval and record the number of reps so you can work to beat your scores when you repeat this workout.

1. Squats
2. Press-ups
3. Chinnies
4. Burpees
5. Skipping - knee lift sprint

EXERCISE DESCRIPTIONS

Squats

You will be performing squats in 30-second intervals during this workout so try to get as many reps as possible completed in each work period. Feel free to use your arms to provide a little extra drive.

- Stand with your feet shoulder-width apart and your hands by your sides.
- Turn your feet out slightly.
- Push your hips back and bend your knees.
- Squat down until your thighs are roughly parallel to the floor.
- Stand back up and repeat.
- Try not to round your lower back at the bottom of the squat as this may lead to injury.

Press-ups

By the fifth set of 30 seconds you may feel you are beginning to find this exercise harder than ever before. Rather than come to a halt, drop to your knees and pump out the reps. It's better to reduce the workload than stop prematurely.

- Bend down and place your hands on the floor, shoulder-width apart. Point your fingers forwards.
- With your arms straight, walk your feet back into the press-up position.
- Check that your heels, hips and shoulders form a straight line.
- Keep your core muscles tight and your neck long – tuck your chin in slightly.
- Bend your elbows and, keeping your arms tucked into your ribs, lower your chest to within 2–3 cm (an inch) of the floor.
- Push back up and return to the starting position.
- If full press-ups are too challenging, bend your legs and place your knees on the floor. This is the three-quarter press-up.
- You can make press-ups more challenging by elevating your feet on a 30–45 cm (12–18 in) high bench.

Chinnies

Chinnies are a traditional ab exercise, used by track and field athletes, that involves spinal flexion and rotation. This is an effective exercise that works your core muscles through multiple planes of movement. As with all sit-up type exercises, do not pull on your head as you may end up hurting your neck.

- Lie on your back with your legs extended and your hands resting on your temples.
- Sit up as you bend and raise your left leg.
- Rotate your upper body and touch your left knee with your right elbow.
- Lie back, extend your leg and return to the starting position and then perform another rep lifting your opposite leg.
- Try to establish a brisk rhythm when performing this exercise.

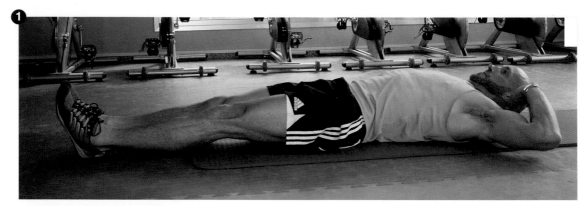

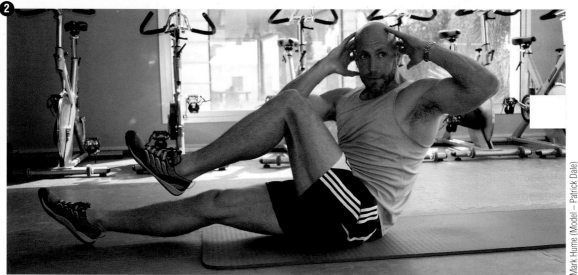

Chinnies – a great
old-school core
exercise

Burpees

If, during the last few sets of this workout, you are finding this exercise tough, feel free to eliminate the press-up or the jump. It's better to keep moving for the duration of the set than grind to a stop. Try to hit the same number of reps each and every set. Remember, pain is only weakness leaving your body!

- Squat down and place your hands on the floor just in front of your feet.
- Jump your feet out behind you so you land in the press-up position.
- Perform a single press-up.
- Jump your feet back under you and up to your hands.
- Leap up into the air as high as you can.
- On landing, immediately drop into another rep.
- Try not to land like a baby elephant when doing this exercise - stay on your toes and, although you are jumping as high as you can, make sure you land as lightly as possible.

Skipping – knee lift sprint

By now, your heart rate will be sky-high and your coordination may be failing you. Dig deep, picture Rocky Balboa in your mind and spin that rope as if you mean it. The higher up you raise your knees, the less likely you are to trip.

- Begin skipping normally and then make a transition to jogging on the spot.
- Keep your body upright and lift your knees so that your thighs are parallel to the floor.
- Pump your legs as fast as you can as you spin your rope.
- This exercise is more challenging – especially if you are new to skipping. Persevere, practise skipping whenever you get the chance and you'll soon be skipping like a pro.

Strength-training Workouts

Strength-training Workout 1

	Exercise	Repetitions	Sets	Recovery	Training system
1	Goblet squats	15–20	2–4	60 seconds	Simple sets
2	Stability ball chest press	15–20	2–4	90 seconds	Super set
3	Body rows	15–20			
4	Alternating lunges	15–20	2–4	60 seconds	Simple sets
5	Seated dumbbell press	15–20	2–4	90 seconds	Super set
6	Lat pull-downs	15–20			
7	Russian twists	15–20	2–4	60 seconds	Simple sets

This workout is designed to increase your basic muscular endurance and teach you some fundamental exercise movement patterns. The exercises selected are purposely simple and the volume relatively low to help 'break you in' to regular strength training. Where you see the term 'super set', perform the paired exercises back-to-back. For example, perform one set of stability ball chest presses and then move immediately on to one set of body rows. Rest for the prescribed time and then repeat the pairing. Simple sets are exactly that; just perform 15-20 reps of the prescribed exercise, rest for 60 seconds and then repeat. With regard to how much weight to use, if you can perform more reps than prescribed the weight is too light, but if you can't manage the lowest number of reps in the range, it's too heavy. Try to either increase the weight or perform more reps on a week-by-week basis.

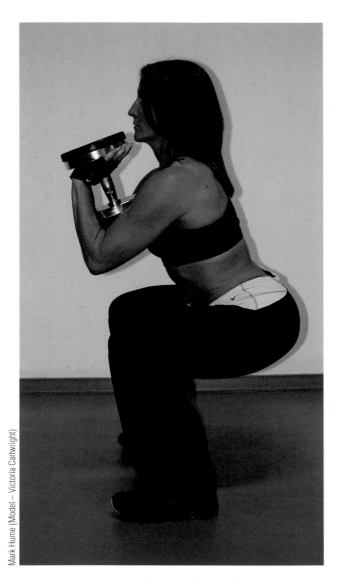

Keep your chest up when performing goblet squats.

EXERCISE DESCRIPTIONS
Goblet squats

Goblet squats target your entire lower body and teach you how to squat properly and safely with weight. If you don't perform this exercise in good form you'll find yourself leaning forwards and potentially dropping the weight. If you notice this happening, you are probably leaning too far forwards, which will cause problems when you move on to more advanced types of squat.

- Perform this exercise with a single dumbbell or kettlebell. You could also perform it with a heavy medicine ball or a big rock!
- Hold your weight in upturned palms and just beneath your chin.
- Make sure your elbows are below your hands and pushed slightly forwards.
- Stand with your feet shoulder-width apart – lift your chest.
- Push your hips back, bend your knees and squat down until your thighs are parallel to the floor.
- Make a conscious effort to push your knees out and lift your chest up.
- Drive down through your heels and stand up.

Stability ball chest press

This exercise will develop coordination, balance and joint stability while targeting your chest, shoulders and triceps muscles. Spending time on this exercise will pay dividends when you move on to other chest exercises such as the bench press. Make sure your stability ball is the right size for you. When sitting on top of the ball with your legs bent and feet flat on the floor, your hips and knees should be level.

- With a dumbbell in each hand, sit carefully on a stability ball.
- Rest the dumbbells on your thighs.
- Walk forwards while simultaneously leaning back on the ball and curling the weights into your armpits.

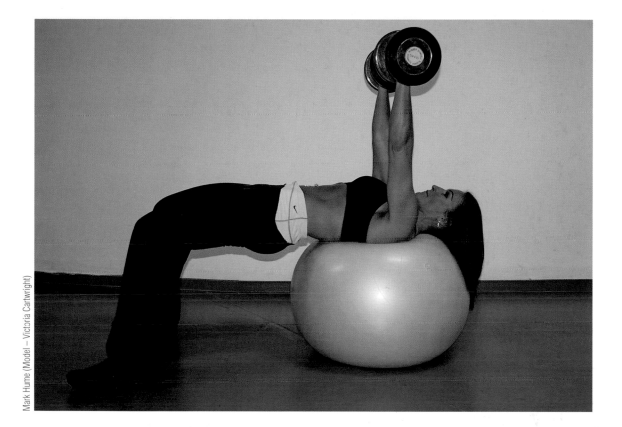

- Position the ball behind your shoulders – your knees should be bent to 90 degrees, your feet flat on the floor and your hips lifted.
- Press the dumbbells over your chest to arms' length.
- Lower the dumbbells back down to your armpits.
- Exhale as you press the weights up and inhale as you lower them.

Stability ball chest presses will develop your coordination and balance.

Body rows

You may have done this exercise before as a substitute for pull-ups. It is an effective upper back and rear shoulder exercise that also challenges your biceps. You can make this exercise more intense by resting a weight across your hips or raising your feet on an exercise bench.

- Adjust the bar on a Smith machine or squat rack to hip-height.
- Sit beneath the bar and grasp it with an overhand shoulder-width grip.
- Extend your legs and lift your butt off the floor – your heels, hips and shoulders should form a straight line.
- Bend your arms and pull your chest up to touch the bar.
- Extend your arms and return to the starting position without bending your knees or hips.

Alternating lunges

Lunges have appeared in various troop phyz workouts, but now you will be performing them while holding dumbbells in your hands or with a barbell across your shoulders. Weighted lunges are much more challenging than the bodyweight version and your balance may not be as solid as it usually is.

- Grasp a dumbbell in each hand, or rest and hold a weight across your upper back.
- Stand with your feet together and your core muscles braced for action.
- Take a large step forwards.
- Bend your legs and lower your rear knee to within 2-3 cm (an inch) of the floor.
- Push off your front leg and spring back to the starting position.
- Perform another rep, leading with your opposite leg.
- Continue alternating legs for the duration of your set.

Using a bench will help support your back and allow you to lift greater weights.

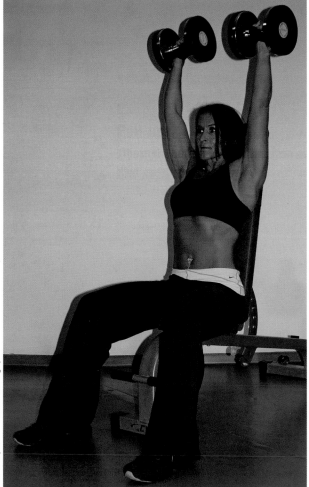

Mark Hume (Model – Victoria Cartwright)

Seated dumbbell press

Pressing weights overhead develops your shoulders and triceps. By performing this exercise in the seated position you can focus purely on driving the weight up. While this does reduce the involvement of your core muscles, it allows you to become familiar with this exercise and provides an essential stepping stone on to more demanding versions of this exercise.

- Position the back rest on an adjustable bench to upright.
- Grasp a dumbbell in each hand and then sit down.
- Lift your chest and arch your lower back slightly.
- Curl the weights up to shoulder height and turn your wrists so your hands are facing forwards.
- Press the dumbbells up and over your head - they should describe a slight arc and come together at arms' length.
- Bend your arms and lower the dumbbells back to shoulder level.

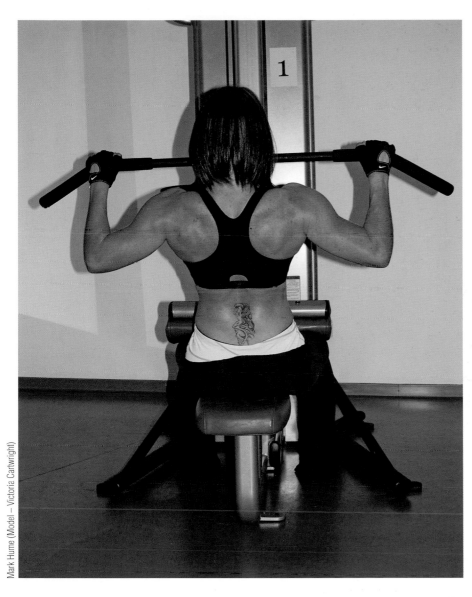

Mark Hume (Model – Victoria Cartwright)

Lat pull-downs are an effective alternative to pull-ups and chin-ups.

Lat pull-downs

Lat pull-downs use the same muscles as pull-ups but the reduced load means that you can perform a higher number of reps – important for developing muscular endurance.

- Grasp the lat pull-down bar with a slightly wider than shoulder-width grip.
- Sit down so that the leg restraints are resting across your thighs.
- With your feet flat on the floor, lean back very slightly and lift your chest.
- Leading with your elbows, pull the bar down to your upper chest.
- Slowly extend your arms and return to the starting position.

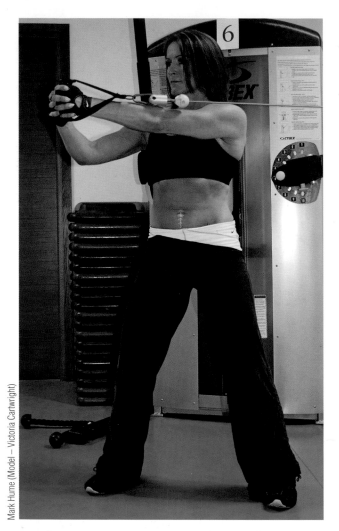

Mark Hume (Model – Victoria Cartwright)

Russian twists

Russian twists target your entire core, with a particular emphasis on your obliques or waist muscles. Don't worry if you find even a light weight very challenging. Most traditional core exercises do not involve resisted rotation and so, in many people, the obliques are woefully underdeveloped. Russian twists are one way to remedy this problem, comrade!

- Stand sideways-on to an adjustable cable machine set to shoulder-height.
- Place your feet shoulder-width apart with your knees slightly bent.
- Grasp the handle with your nearest hand and then place your other hand on top.
- Keeping your feet still, your hands aligned with the centre of your chest and your arms just shy of fully extended, rotate your upper body through 180 degrees.
- Imagine your upper body is a tank turret and your legs are the tracks. Try to turn your upper body independently of your legs.
- Slowly return to the starting position and repeat. On completion, perform this exercise on the opposite side.

Russian Twists – this unusually named exercise targets your oblique or waist muscles.

Strength-training Workout 2

Strength-training Workout 2 builds on the foundations established in the previous workout and is designed to increase your muscle size. The exercises selected for this workout are slightly more complex than those performed in Workout 1, but you are now ready for a greater challenge. This workout utilizes a training system called Escalating Density Training (EDT for short). EDT is a non-traditional way of designing a workout but it is very effective for muscle building. Simply attempt to perform as many reps as possible of each paired exercise in the given time. For example, perform a set of incline dumbbell bench presses and then a set of bent-over dumbbell rows. Move back and forth, taking as little rest as possible, to clock up as many reps as possible (designated as AMRAP in the workout) in the allotted time. Make a note of your total reps and try to beat that total next time.

	Exercise	Repetitions	Sets	Recovery	Training system
1	Front squats	8–12	3–4	90 seconds	Pyramid
2	Incline dumbbell bench press	8–12	AMRAP in 15 Minutes		Escalating density training
3	Bent-over dumbbell rows	8–12			
4	Bulgarian split squats	8–12	3–4	60 seconds	Simple sets
5	Standing barbell press	8–12	AMRAP in 10 Minutes		Escalating density training
6	Chin-ups (supinated grip)	8–12			
7	Cable wood chop	8–12	3–4	90 seconds	Simple sets

EXERCISE DESCRIPTIONS

Front squats

Front squats are similar to goblet squats in that they develop your entire lower body. However, the position of the bar makes this version of the ever-effective squat much more challenging and allows for a heavier weight to be used. You'll need a barbell for this exercise.

Thrust your elbows forwards when performing front squats.

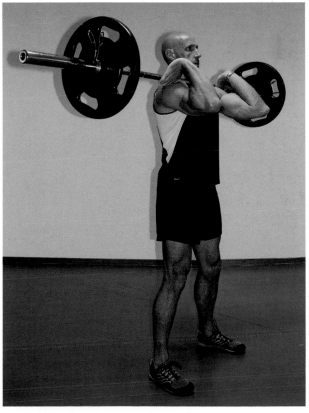

- Place a barbell in a squat rack at just below shoulder level.
- Grasp the barbell with a shoulder-width overhand grip.
- Roll your elbows under the bar and then rack the barbell across your anterior (front) deltoids.
- Lift the bar out of the rack and step back.
- Position your feet shoulder-width apart, lift your chest and thrust your elbows forwards.
- Push your hips back, bend your knees and squat down until your thighs are at least parallel to the floor.
- Drive down through your heels and stand back up.
- Make a conscious effort to keep your elbows pointing directly forwards at all times and do not allow your lower back to round.

Mark Hume (Model – Patrick Dale)

Incline dumbbell bench press

Incline dumbbell presses target your upper chest, shoulders and triceps.

Incline dumbbell bench presses target the upper or clavicular part of your chest as well as your shoulders and triceps. If you don't have access to an adjustable bench, you can simply raise one end of your bench on an exercise step, a stack of weight plates or even some bricks.

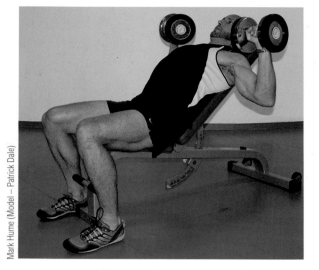

- Set the back rest on an adjustable bench to around 30 degrees.
- Grasp a dumbbell in each hand and sit down.
- Lean back and simultaneously raise the dumbbells up to your shoulders.
- Rotate your wrists so that your palms are facing forwards.
- Lift your chest and arch your lower back slightly.
- Exhale and press the weights up and directly over your shoulders.
- Inhale and lower the dumbbells back to your shoulders.
- Repeat for the prescribed number of reps.

Bent-over dumbbell rows

Bent-over dumbbell rows. Keep your chest lifted and your core tight when you perform this exercise.

This exercise targets your lats, upper back muscles and biceps. It's less technically demanding than body rows but the supported, one-armed action employed in this exercise means that you can use a heavier weight in relative safety.

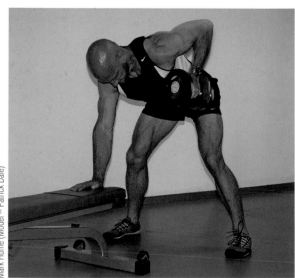

- Grasp a dumbbell in one hand and stand with your knees slightly bent.
- Lean forwards from your hips and rest your opposite hand on a knee-high bench.
- Let your arm hang straight down from your shoulder but do not relax – keep your shoulder pulled back in its socket.
- Keeping your upper body still and without flexing your legs, pull the dumbbell up and into your upper ribs. Make sure you lead with your elbow.
- Slowly extend your arm and return to the starting position.
- Perform the prescribed number of reps and then change arms.

Bulgarian split squats

An unusually named exercise that will challenge your mobility, strength and balance. Some strength coaches suggest that the Bulgarian split squat is one of the most effective leg-developing exercises you can do. Whether this is true or not, it is certainly a great movement that will increase your leg strength, one limb at a time.

The Bulgarian split squat. Requiring flexibility and balance, this unusually named exercise is a great leg developer.

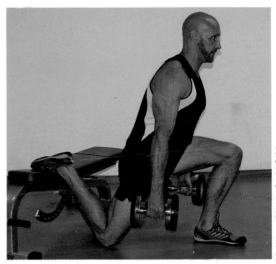

- Stand with your back to a knee-high bench.
- Grasp a dumbbell in each hand and bend one leg so that it rests on top of the bench behind you.
- Hop forwards until you are in a comfortable 'split' stance.
- Bend your legs and lower your rear knee as far down towards the floor as is comfortable.
- Make sure you keep your torso upright at all times.
- Stand back up and then repeat. Perform the prescribed number of reps and then change legs.
- You can also perform this exercise with a barbell across your shoulders.

Standing barbell press

Commonly referred to as the military press, this exercise challenges your shoulders, triceps and core muscles. Old-school strongmen used to prize this exercise above all others and pressing weights overhead was once one of the Olympic lifts. Bench presses have replaced the military press as most people's favourite exercise, but the reality is that this exercise offers a far greater functional carry-over than an exercise you perform on your back!

The military press – performed by soldiers the world over

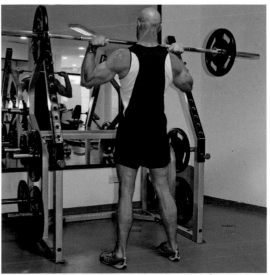

- Place a barbell in a squat rack at just below shoulder height.
- Grasp the barbell with a shoulder-width over-hand grip.
- With your elbows below your hands and the bar resting on your shoulders, lift the barbell from the rack.
- Step back slightly and then stand with your feet shoulder-width apart and your knees slightly bent.
- Brace your core muscles to support your spine.

- Without using your legs, press the barbell directly over your head to arms' length.
- Lower the bar back to your shoulders and repeat.

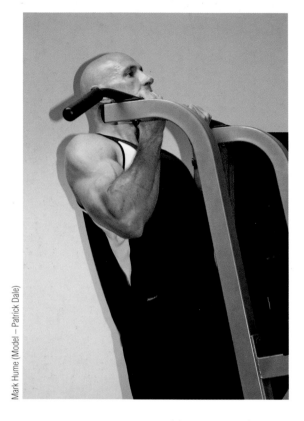

Chin-ups (supinated grip)

Up to now you have performed pull-ups. Why? Because pull-ups are harder! Chin-ups place your biceps in a superior pulling angle, which means that you should be able to perform this exercise either for more reps or with weight attached to your waist. Also, chin-ups are a superior biceps building exercise and every soldier wants to have big guns! (Guns – used to describe weapons and also your arms.)

- Grasp the pull-up bar with an underhand, slightly narrower than shoulder-width grip.
- Hang at full stretch with your arms fully extended and your feet clear of the floor.
- Bend your arms and pull your chin up and over the bar.
- Slowly straighten your arms to return to the starting position.
- If you are unable to perform chin-ups, substitute underhand grip lat pulls-downs.

The supinated grip used in chin-ups makes them slightly easier than pull-ups!

Cable wood chop

Resisted rotation exercises don't come much more effective than cable wood chops. The high to low action combined with shifting your weight from one leg to the other really taxes your entire core and also teaches you to integrate your upper and lower body into a single, synergistic unit.

- Stand sideways-on to an adjustable cable machine set to head-height.
- Position your feet two shoulder-widths apart.
- Grasp the handle with your nearest hand and then place your other hand on top.
- Shift your weight over towards the weight stack. This position should resemble a sideways lunge with one leg bent and the other straight.
- Keeping your feet still, your hands aligned with the centre of your chest and your arms just shy of fully extended, rotate your upper body through 180 degrees as you simultaneously shift your weight across to your other leg.
- Slowly return to the starting position and repeat. On completion, perform this exercise on the opposite side.

Military Fitness

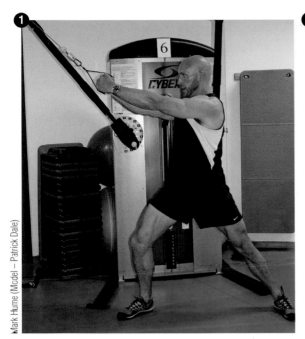
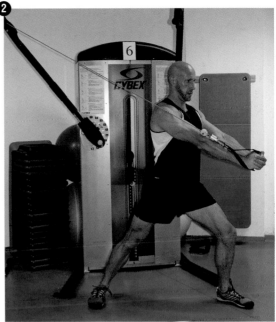

Mark Hume (Model – Patrick Dale)

The cable wood chop – focus on turning your arms, shoulders and head all together – just like a tank turret!

Strength-training Workout 3

	Exercise	Repetitions	Sets	Recovery	Training System
1	Back squats	4–6			
2	Barbell bench press	4–6	4–5	90 seconds	Tri set
3	Wrestler's row	4–6			
4	Split squat jumps	4–6			
5	Standing alternating dumbbell press	4–6	4–5	90 seconds	Tri set
6	Pull-ups (pronated grip)	4–6			
7	Turkish get up	4–6	4–5	60 seconds	Simple sets

Strength-training workout 3 focuses on building your basic strength by using heavier weights and fewer reps. It is common to rest for up to 3 minutes between sets when training for strength, but this is hardly practical. Soldiers use the term 'concurrent activity' to describe doing two or more things at once and that is a technique employed in this workout. Instead of sitting and resting for 3 minutes, just go and perform your second and then your third exercise. Don't rush though – remember you are merely making the most of your time rather than trying to challenge your cardiovascular system.

EXERCISE DESCRIPTIONS

Back squats

Back squats are one of the most effective exercises that you can perform to increase your lower body strength. The position of the bar allows you to support a significant amount of weight and also forces you to use your glutes, lower back and hamstrings very strongly to maintain an upright body position. Perform this exercise in a squat rack for safety. Although you can perform your squats using a Smith machine, this is not recommended as, although a Smith machine will prevent you from dropping the weight, it also means that the bar cannot travel through its normal trajectory and therefore places an undue strain on your knees, hips and lower back.

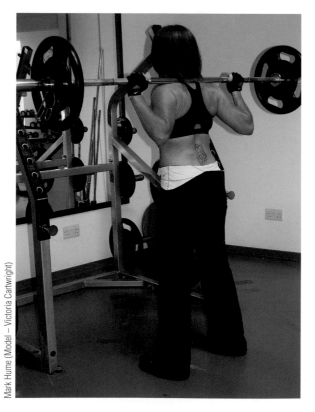

Mark Hume (Model – Victoria Cartwright)

- Place a barbell in a squat rack at just below shoulder height.
- Grasp the bar with a slightly wider than shoulder-width grip and then duck under the bar.
- Press the fleshy upper portion of your back against the bar.
- Grip the bar tightly and pull it down on to your upper back.
- Lift the weight off the rack pins and take a step back.
- Stand with your feet shoulder-width apart and your toes turned slightly outwards.
- Lift your chest and push your elbows forwards.
- Push your hips back, bend your knees and squat down until your thighs are parallel to the floor.
- Drive down through your heels and stand back up.
- Do not allow your lower back to become rounded.

Back squats – lead with your hips and keep your chest lifted.

Barbell bench press

This classic test of upper body strength will develop your chest, shoulders and triceps. Always perform the bench press with a spotter or in a power rack as, if you miss a lift, you can end up with a heavy barbell across your chest and no means to escape from beneath it. Needless to say, this can cause very serious injury. If you don't have access to a power rack or a spotter, perform bench presses using dumbbells instead.

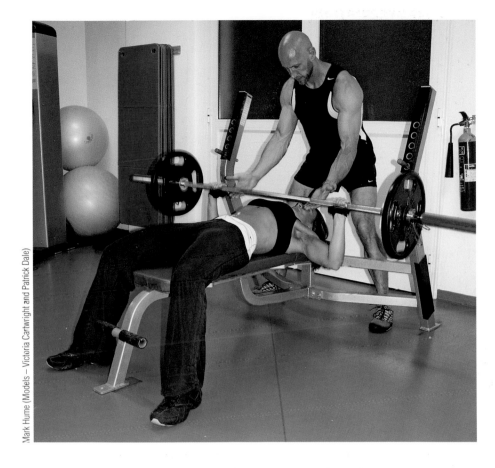

Mark Hume (Models – Victoria Cartwright and Patrick Dale)

Always use a spotter when bench pressing.

- Lie on your back with your eyes directly below the barbell.
- Plant your feet firmly on the floor and arch your lower back slightly.
- Grasp the barbell with an overhand, slightly wider than shoulder-width, grip.
- Unrack the bar and hold it directly over your shoulders.
- Bend your arms and lower the bar to within 2–3 cm (an inch) of the highest part of your chest.
- Drive it back up to arms' length.
- Do not move your feet or head at any time during your lift.

Wrestler's row

The wrestler's row is a challenging exercise that will develop your entire back as well as your glutes and leg muscles. Focus on maintaining good posture and don't be surprised that even relatively light weights provide a very demanding workout.

- Grasp a dumbbell or kettlebell in each hand.
- Stand with your feet hip-width apart, your knees slightly bent and your hands by your sides.

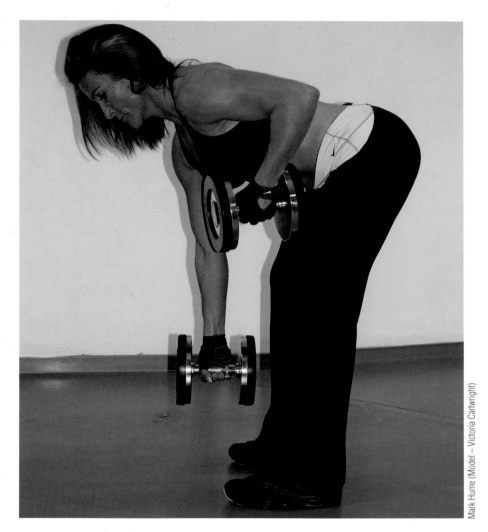

Wrestler's row – bend your knees, arch your back slightly and keep one elbow tucked into your ribs at all times!

Mark Hume (Model – Victoria Cartwright)

- Bend forwards from your hips.
- Bend both arms and pull the dumbbells into your armpits and hold them there - this is your starting position.
- Keeping your chest lifted and avoiding rounding your back, lower one dumbbell towards the floor - when your arm reaches full extension, pull it back into your body.
- Perform a second rep with your opposite arm.
- Continue alternating arms until your set is complete.

Split squat jumps

This lunge variation will develop explosive leg power, which will translate to faster running and higher jumping. Technically a plyometric exercise, you should try to minimize ground contact time when performing it.

Military Fitness

- Stand with your feet together and your hands by your sides.
- Take a large step forwards and bend your legs – lower your rear knee to within 2-3 cm (an inch) of the floor.
- Jump up into the air and swing your rear leg forwards and your front leg backwards.
- Land and bend your legs, immediately preparing for another jump.
- Continue jumping and switching legs for the prescribed number of reps.
- Be careful not to let your rear knee hit the floor – bruised knees are not a good look!

Standing alternating dumbbell press

This final overhead pressing variation will challenge your balance, coordination and core strength. Although the increased complexity of this exercise may necessitate lighter weights than usual, this is more than made up for by the increased time your muscles will spend under load and the additional challenge of balancing the dumbbells.

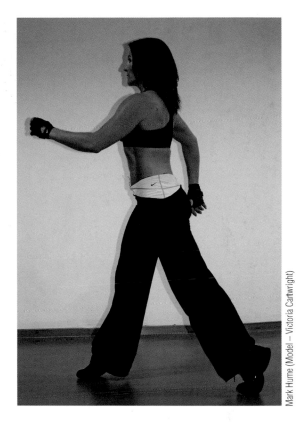

Mark Hume (Model – Victoria Cartwright)

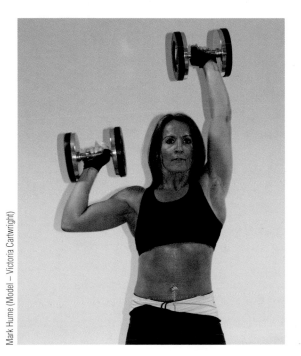

Mark Hume (Model – Victoria Cartwright)

- Grasp a dumbbell in each hand and stand with your feet shoulder-width apart.
- Curl the dumbbells up to shoulder level.
- Turn your wrists to face forwards.
- Hold one arm steady as you press the opposite dumbbell up and overhead to arm's length.
- Lower this dumbbell back to your shoulder and then press the other dumbbell up.
- Continue alternating arms for the duration of your set.

Split squat jumps – jump as high as you can and get lots of hang-time!

Brace your abs to support your spine when performing these dumbbell presses.

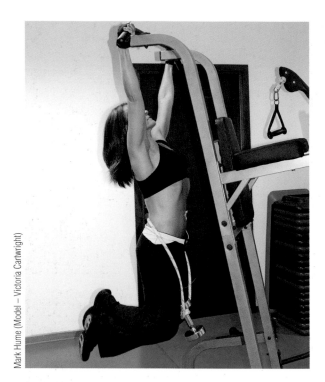

Mark Hume (Model – Victoria Cartwright)

Pull-ups (pronated grip)

You are more than familiar with pull-ups now, but as you are performing this exercise for strength and not muscular endurance, you may well need to attach weights around your waist to make it sufficiently challenging.

- Grasp an overhead bar with a slightly wider than shoulder-width overhand grip.
- Hang at full stretch with your arms and legs extended – this is called the dead hang position.
- Pull strongly with your arms and lift your chin up and over the bar.
- Slowly lower to the starting position and repeat.
- If you are unable to do pull-ups, perform lat pull-downs with an overhand slightly wider than shoulder-width grip instead.

Fix a weight around your waist to make this pull-up exercise more demanding.

Turkish get up

This oddly named exercise is one of the most effective total-body and core movements around. Traditionally performed with a kettlebell, you can also use a dumbbell, medicine ball or even a barbell for resistance. Use a light weight initially, maybe even just a token 2–5 kg (5–11 lb), until you are familiar and comfortable with this excellent exercise.

- Lie on your back with your legs straight and holding a single weight with your left arm, extended straight up and perpendicular to the floor.
- Bend your left leg and place your foot as close to your butt as you can.
- Rest your right arm on the floor about 45 cm (18 in) from your side with your palm turned down.
- Push down through your left foot and your right hand and roll over on to your right butt cheek.
- 'Punch' the dumbbell away as you sit up. Remember to keep your arm perpendicular to the floor.
- Lift your hips off the floor and then step back with your right leg so that you can place your knee on the floor – you should now be in a kneeling lunge position.
- Slowly stand up while ensuring your arm remains aloft.
- Reverse this sequence of moves to return to the floor.
- Perform for the prescribed number of reps and then swap sides.

Opposite
Whether this exercise originated in Turkey or not, it is an awesome core conditioner!

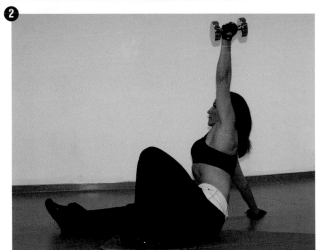

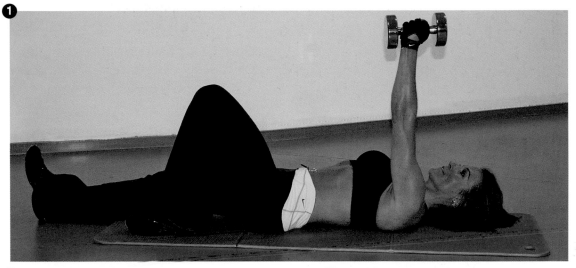

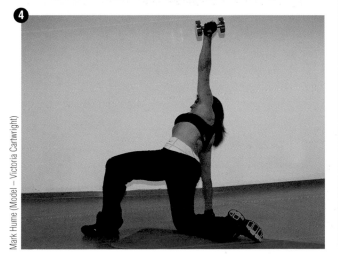

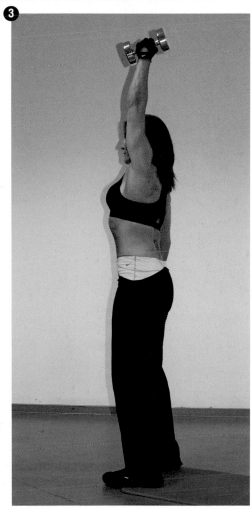

Mark Hume (Model – Victoria Cartwright)

Twice-weekly Strength Training

If you are an intermediate to advanced strength-trainer, you may want to lift weights more than once a week. In fact, if you are lifting particularly heavy weights, this may actually be a necessity, as you might find that you are too tired by the middle to end of your strength workout to do much justice to the lifts later in the programme.

Remember that the focus of this programme is developing functional strength and so training with weights twice a week is not an opportunity to do a whole lot of extra sets and reps in pursuit of muscle hypertrophy. The point of 'abbreviating' the Magnificent Seven strength-training routine is to increase the *quality* of the work performed, not the *quantity*. An intermediate or advanced lifter who trains with heavy weights will tire more quickly and require longer rests between sets and, by eliminating some of the exercises from the standard once-a-week routine, you have more time to focus on fewer key exercises.

For intermediate/advanced lifters, I suggest the following weekly template.

Monday	Tuesday	Wednesday	Thursday	Friday	Saturday	Sunday
Troop phyz	Strength workout A	Boot run	Troop phyz	Strength workout B	Yomp	Rest

Strength Workout A

	Exercise	Repetitions	Sets	Recovery
1	Back squats	10, 8, 6, 6, 6	5	90–180 seconds
2	Barbell bench press	10, 8, 6, 6, 6	5	90–180 seconds
3	Bent-over dumbbell rows	10, 8, 6, 6, 6	5	60–90 seconds
4	Russian twists	12, 10, 8, 8, 8	5	60–90 seconds

EXERCISE DESCRIPTIONS
Back squats

As the champion lower body strengthening exercise, no abbreviated strength workout would be complete without squats. Remember to keep your chest up and your core tight and drive down through your heels. Power lifters say that 'shallow squats are useless squats', so try to break parallel with your thighs on each and every rep to get the most from this super-effective exercise.

- Place a barbell in a squat rack at just below shoulder height.
- Grasp the bar with a slightly wider than shoulder-width grip and then duck under the bar.
- Press the fleshy upper portion of your back against the bar.
- Grip the bar tightly and pull it down on to your upper back.
- Lift the weight and take a step back.
- Stand with your feet shoulder-width apart and your toes turned slightly outwards.
- Lift your chest and push your elbows forwards.
- Push your hips back, bend your knees and squat down until your thighs are parallel to the floor.
- Drive down through your heels and stand back up.
- Do not allow your lower back to become rounded.

Barbell bench press

Bench presses build prodigious pushing strength in your chest, shoulders and arms, but they are also an 'ego lift' for many people. They hoist and bounce and jerk the bar up and down with little or no thought to the muscles involved in this superior upper body builder. Lower the bar under control, lightly touch the bar to your chest, pause for a split second and then drive the bar up and off your chest to full arm extension. Technique is everything in the bench press – both to make the exercise as effective as possible and also to limit injury potential.

- Lie on your back with your eyes directly below the barbell.
- Plant your feet firmly on the floor and arch your lower back slightly.
- Grasp the barbell with an overhand grip, slightly wider than shoulder-width.
- Unrack the bar and hold it directly over your shoulders.
- Bend your arms and lower the bar to within 2–3 cm (an inch) of the highest part of your chest.
- Drive it back up to arms' length.
- Do not move your feet or head at any time during your lift.

Bent-over dumbbell rows

Your lower back may well be fatigued after squats, so this supported pulling exercise allows you to really focus on your back muscles without having to worry too much about your spine. That doesn't mean you can use sloppy technique – keep your chest lifted, your lower back slightly arched and your abs tight, as failure to do so could still result in injury.

- Grasp a dumbbell in one hand and stand with your knees slightly bent.
- Lean forwards from your hips and rest your opposite hand on a knee-high bench.

- Let your arm hang straight down from your shoulder but do not relax – keep your shoulder pulled back in its socket.
- Keeping your upper body still, and without flexing your legs, pull the dumbbell up and into your upper ribs. Makes sure you lead with your elbow.
- Slowly extend your arm and return to the starting position.
- Perform the prescribed number of reps and then change arms.

Russian twists

Rotational movements are seldom performed by most trainees. This is a shame as not only do well-developed obliques add to your core strength and spinal health, they also contribute to the appearance of your entire midsection. Think of your obliques as the muscles that frame your abdominals. You wouldn't display an amazing piece of art without a frame, so don't leave your abs without well-developed obliques!

- Stand sideways-on to an adjustable cable machine set to shoulder-height.
- Place your feet shoulder-width apart, with your knees slightly bent.
- Grasp the handle with your nearest hand and then place your other hand on top.
- Keeping your feet still, your hands aligned with the centre of your chest and your arms just shy of fully extended, rotate your upper body through 180 degrees.
- Imagine your upper body is a tank turret and your legs are the tracks. Try to turn your upper body independently of your legs.
- Slowly return to the starting position and repeat. On completion, perform this exercise on the opposite side.

Strength Workout B

	Exercise	Repetitions	Sets	Recovery
1	Dead lifts	10, 8, 6, 6, 6	5	90–180 seconds
2	Standing barbell press	10, 8, 6, 6, 6	5	90–180 seconds
3	Chin-ups	10, 8, 6, 6, 6	5	60–90 seconds
4	Ab wheel roll-out	10, 10, 10, 10, 10	5	60–90 seconds

Dead lifts

If squats are the kings of the exercise royal family then dead lifts are the queens with aspirations to overthrow the kings! Dead lifts are an excellent posterior chain exercise; they target all of the muscles on the back of your body from your heels to the base of your skull. They also strengthen your upper back, core and forearms. Good technique is essential when you perform dead lifts as rounding your back or letting your hips rise too quickly can place a significant and potentially injurious load on your lower back.

- With a barbell on the floor, stand with your feet hip-width apart and your toes beneath the bar.
- Bend down and grasp the bar with an overhand shoulder-width grip. Extend your arms, lift your chest and drop your hips below your shoulders. Your shoulders should be directly over the bar.
- Drive your feet into the floor, extend your legs and hips and stand up.
- Once erect, hold this position for a second and then push your hips back, bend your knees and lower the bar back to the floor.
- Check and reset your position and repeat.
- Exhale as you are lowering the bar and inhale as you lift it.
- Do not allow your lower back to become rounded or your hips to rise faster than your shoulders as this can lead to serious injury.

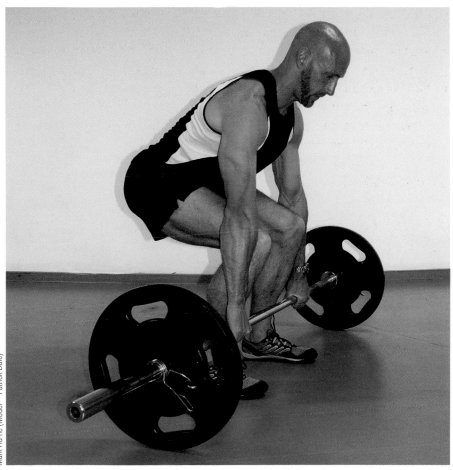

Mark Hume (Model – Patrick Dale)

Dead lifts - a great total-body exercise!

Standing barbell press

Before bench pressing became the most popular exercise seen in gyms, the overhead standing press was the exercise by which strongmen measured their lifting ability. Back in the good old days, there were no such things as exercise benches. All exercises were performed in the standing position and that was that. The physiques of the old-time strong men reflected their love of hoisting massive loads overhead and huge, well-rounded shoulders and thick triceps were all the rage. Overhead lifting also strengthens your core and even your legs – something that can't be said of the bench press.

- Place a barbell in a squat rack at just below shoulder height.
- Grasp the barbell with a shoulder-width overhand grip.
- With your elbows below your hands and the bar resting on your shoulders, lift the barbell from the rack.
- Step back slightly and then stand with your feet shoulder-width apart and your knees slightly bent.
- Brace your core muscles to support your spine.
- Without using your legs, press the barbell directly over your head to arms' length.
- Lower the bar back to your shoulders and repeat.

Chin-ups (supinated grip)

Chin-ups really work your biceps hard, despite technically being an upper back exercise. Focus on gripping the bar as hard as you can and driving your elbows down and back to get the most from this exercise. Add weight set by set to keep you within the prescribed range of reps – the last rep of each set should be really tough to complete.

- Grasp the pull-up bar with a slightly narrower than shoulder-width grip.
- Hang at full stretch, with your arms fully extended and your feet clear of the floor.
- Bend your arms and pull your chin up and over the bar.
- Slowly straighten your arms to return to the starting position.
- If you are unable to perform chin-ups, substitute under hand grip lat pull-downs.

Ab wheel roll-outs

Performed with an ab wheel or a loaded barbell, the roll-out is a tough but effective exercise that strengthens your rectus abdominis muscle. Rectus abdominis, abs for short and essentially your six-pack, must work very hard to stabilize your spine during this challenging movement. Start off by performing this exercise on your knees and progress to the standing version only when you are able to perform 12–15 perfect kneeling reps.

- Kneel on the floor with the ab wheel or barbell close to your legs.
- Keep your arms straight throughout this exercise.
- Inhale, brace your abs and push the wheel/barbell along the floor away from you.
- Extend your hips as far as you can to lower your head and chest towards the floor.
- Pause in the most stretched position you can maintain.
- Exhale, lift your hips and pull the wheel/barbell back to your legs.
- Continue for the desired number of reps.
- If you feel any discomfort in your lower back when performing this exercise, check that you are not overextending your lower back and consider reducing your range of movement until your strength increases.
- Once you are proficient at performing the kneeling version of this exercise, try doing it from a standing position. Initially only roll the wheel/barbell out as far as your shoulders. Gradually increase the length of your roll as you get stronger.

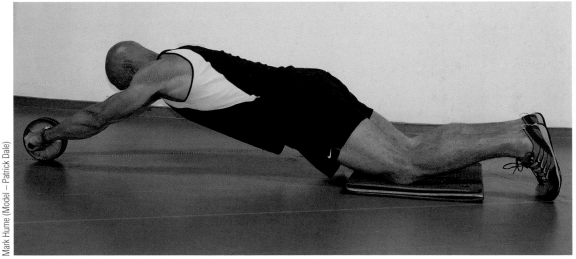

Every squaddie loves equipment and gadgets and in the following chapter you'll find a list of items that may help to make your training more enjoyable and productive, or simply save you having to join a gym!

Performed with an ab wheel or a barbell, ab wheel roll-outs work your core muscles hard.

CHAPTER SIX

Equipment Options

A trip to the Quartermaster's store

As discussed previously, military fitness training is not reliant on fancy exercise equipment. Soldiers can usually find a way of turning almost anything into a workout tool. Got no weights? Use a water-filled jerry-can. No dumbbells? Ammo boxes filled with sand will suffice. No medicine balls available? Sandbags are an excellent substitute. Military fitness training is very much a case of 'improvise, adapt and overcome' and a lack of training equipment is no reason to miss workouts.

Many of the troop phyz workouts are completely equipment-free, so you can perform these training sessions just about anywhere. Most of them were designed when I was serving onboard a ship and had nothing more than a space on the upper deck and a beam from which to perform pull-ups. I was limited to whatever training equipment I could carry in my Bergen (rucksack) and that inevitably meant that a skipping rope was all I could muster. Despite being confined to a ship for long periods of time, I not only managed to stay fit, I actually got fitter, stronger and leaner as a result of these 'stripped down' workouts.

Your body is an absolutely amazing organism that can detect and respond to dozens of stimuli and perform phenomenal feats of strength and endurance, as well as providing housing and transportation for one of the most advanced computers ever – your brain, in case you were wondering. However, in some ways, your body is also as dumb as a bag of spanners! It has no idea if you are performing press-ups on the deck of a grimy Royal Navy ship in the middle of the Mediterranean Sea or performing dumbbell chest presses in a state-of-the-art gym at your local health and fitness emporium. All your body knows is tension and overload. If sufficient overload is applied and there are enough resources available for recovery, your body will get fitter. We will discuss the importance of nutrition in the next chapter, but for now we will focus on some low-tech equipment options that you can use to develop your fitness.

Considerations

This section is not meant to be exhaustive but, rather, to give you a few ideas of how you can get as fit as possible without having to resort to joining a gym or spending lots of money. To make it onto this list, the training tools listed had to meet a number of criteria:

- Low cost – fitness training should not be financially exclusive.
- Practical – items should be easily available.
- Versatile – the more uses for a particular item, the better.
- Combat tested – any tools listed have been used 'in the field' and proved their effectiveness.
- Safe – minimal risk of injury.

Sandbags

Sandbags provide an excellent alternative to barbells, dumbbells and kettlebells. In some ways they are actually better as, when you lift them, the sand shifts and results in increased recruitment of your core and joint stabilizing muscles. On the downside, unless you have a set of scales to hand, it can be hard to quantify the exact weight of your sandbags – although if you make the version detailed below, this is not really an issue.

To make a set of sandbag weights you'll need the following:

1. Large quantity of sand, gravel or similar
2. Big plastic beaker
3. Heavy duty zip-lock bags
4. Strong parcel tape
5. Kitchen scales
6. A large seaman's kit bag or ex-army duffel bag

Fill your large plastic beaker with sand and weigh it – make a note of how heavy it is. This will save you weighing each sandbag weight you make.

Take a zip-lock bag and fill it with sand. Don't fill it completely as this will increase the chances that it will split during use. Make sure it weighs a nice round number, for example 2 kg or 5 lb, as this will make it easier to calculate how much weight you are lifting. Squeeze the air out of the bag and zip it up. Place this bag inside another and then seal it shut using the parcel tape. Wrap the bag in tape to strengthen it and minimize the risk of leaks. Repeat this process until you have made as many sandbag weights as you need. It's a good idea to make a few different sizes based on multiples of your initial weight that can then be mixed and matched according to the exercise you are performing.

Once you have manufactured your sandbag weights you simply load them into your duffel bag, tie off the neck and get started with your workout. Add or remove sandbag weights as necessary. It's better to grip the material of the sandbag rather than making use of any of the built-in handles as, in the first place, the handles sometimes rip off and secondly, by gripping the bag, you will strengthen your forearms and hands much more effectively. Personally, I would cut the handles off to avoid the temptation to use them.

Even though you have double-bagged your sand and each bag is housed inside a sturdy duffel bag, the sand can still leak out. This is less of a problem with coarser gravel, but fine sand has an unerring ability to get everywhere – just ask any squaddie who has served in the desert! Because of this, sandbags are best suited to outdoor use or, at the very least, an area with hard floors from which any spillage can easily be swept.

If you prefer, you can buy a commercially manufactured exercise sandbag kit. There are a number of excellent products available which are generally leak-proof and come supplied with an outer shell, super-tough zip-lock bags and an instruction manual or DVD. Other than being more leak-proof, these products are not really any more effective than the virtually free version detailed above but, if you'd rather have a Rolls-Royce than an old Land Rover, one of these kits is worth considering.

Sledgehammers

Most exercisers enjoy hitting things and this is especially true of soldiers. It's a throwback to your hunter-gatherer days and also appeals to that mostly dormant lizard part of your brain. For whatever reason, bashing the living hell out of an inanimate object is just plain fun! It's also fantastic exercise. A punch bag is a great piece of exercise equipment but free-standing bags are expensive and regular bags need sturdy, permanent mountings, so it's not always practical to have a punch bag in your home. Luckily, there is a cheap alternative readily available to allow you to get your fix of hitting stuff – a sledgehammer.

Swinging a sledgehammer is a great full-body exercise – there is barely a muscle that isn't involved. You can use a sledgehammer to develop muscle power by performing short, hard sets of swings, or cardiovascular fitness and muscular endurance by performing longer, less forceful sets. Sledgehammer training is a popular workout with some of the toughest and fittest athletes on the planet – mixed martial arts fighters. And if it's good enough for them, it'll be good enough for you!

A sledgehammer, tyre and gloves make for a low-tech but highly effective workout!

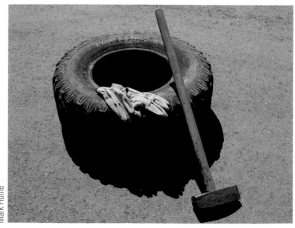

Mark Hume

Sledgehammers are available in a wide range of weights. Don't think you have to get the heaviest one you can find though – you want a hammer that will allow you to generate maximum force. Too light and there will be next to no training effect, but too heavy and you won't be able to swing it effectively. Personally, I use a 5.5 kg (12 pound) hammer and that seems just right for the majority of my workouts. There is no need to buy a specialist strength-training sledgehammer – just buy a basic model from your local DIY superstore. You'll also need a pair of work gloves to protect your hands.

Military Fitness

Most proponents of sledgehammer training favour an old SUV tyre as a striking target. You can probably pick one up free from your local tyre depot. Lay the tyre on its side and aim your hammer at its wall. The wall will absorb the shock of the hammer strike and also provides a bit of recoil, which will help you establish a good swinging rhythm. A tyre is ideal if you intend to use your hammer in your garage or on your patio as it effectively protects the surface below. I don't recommend you try this indoors though ...

You can also use an old tree stump, log, sandpit or dirt patch as your striking target, but a tyre is by far the best option.

Swinging Techniques

Swinging a sledgehammer isn't technically demanding but it does require some coordination. It's important to have sound technique before getting too gung ho with your hammer otherwise there is a possibility of serious self-inflicted injury. There are a number of gripping options for you to experiment with. The 'no choke' method, where you grip the hammer handle near the end, is probably the most demanding, but that doesn't mean it's always the best. Make sure you swing your hammer using both left and right hand leading grips to avoid developing muscle imbalances.

Experiment with your stance – some users prefer a squared-off stance while others are more comfortable in a staggered or split stance. If you use a split stance, remember to alternate your leading leg as you change hands. The standard sledgehammer grips and swinging techniques are:

If you are going to hit it, then hit it hard!

- 'Choked' grip – your uppermost hand slides up and down the handle as you swing the hammer.
- Left hand lead – your left hand is above your right.
- Right hand lead – your right hand is above your left.
- Alternating hands – change leading hand swing by swing.
- 'No choke' grip – you hold the hammer by the end and your hands do not move.

Sledgehammer Workouts

There are a number of workouts that you can perform with your sledgehammer and these are just a few of my favourites. If you want to incorporate sledgehammer training into your workouts try performing some swings as a 'finisher' to your strength-training workouts or as an addition/replacement to some of the troop phyz workouts.

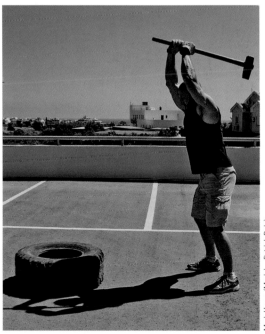

Mark Hume (Model – Patrick Dale)

Timed intervals

Decide on a work-to-rest ratio (e.g. 2 minutes of work, 1 minute of rest) and repeat for the desired number of sets. One of my favourite interval schemes is 3 minutes of striking (left hand on top), rest 1 minute, 3 minutes of striking (right hand on top), rest 1 minute, 3 minutes of alternating hand on top. This scheme provides a great finish to a regular workout and is a nice stand-alone mini workout when time is short. No matter what set/rep scheme you select, just make sure you work really hard during the 'on' periods and you'll find interval training a very effective, time-efficient training method.

The duration of your work/rest intervals is very much goal dependent:
- Shorter sets, e.g. less than 20 seconds, are excellent for developing maximum force and therefore increasing muscle power.
- Medium-length sets, e.g. 45–90 seconds, are ideal for improving muscular endurance and anaerobic conditioning.
- Longer sets, e.g. 2 minutes and above, are best suited to the development of aerobic fitness and muscular endurance.

Tabata intervals

As discussed in Chapter 3, the Tabata Method involves performing 8–10 sets of very high-intensity exercise of 20 seconds' duration, separated by 10-second recovery periods, giving a total training time of 4–5 minutes. The caveat of the Tabata Method is that all the intervals have to be performed at 100% intensity – an absolute flat-out effort. You have to strive to perform as much work in each 20-second interval as possible and try to maintain that work rate for all of the 8–10 sets. The old adage that you can train long and easy, or short and hard, has never been truer than when describing the Tabata Method! As with any type of exercise, the Tabata Method should be preceded by an appropriate warm-up of 5–10 minutes and followed by a cool-down of similar duration. All in all the session could take as little as 15 minutes – perfect if you are short on time but still want great results from your training. I once used Tabata sledgehammer training as my sole form of cardiovascular exercise for a month and found that I lost fat, gained fitness and also got significantly more powerful – all from two 10-minute workouts a week!

Repetition intervals

With this system, instead of using time as your measure of work, you'll be using reps instead. For example you may do 20 strikes and then rest for 30 seconds and repeat for as many sets as desired. Another one of my favourite sessions involves doing 20 strikes every minute for 10–15 minutes. Each set takes between 35 and 45 seconds, leaving 15–25 seconds to rest before I start the next set. The beauty of sets starting on the minute is that you just need to be able to see the sweep hand of a clock, so there is no need to push buttons or programme intervals into a stopwatch.

Timed density blocks

Allocate a time block (e.g. 5 or 10 minutes) and aim to perform as many strikes as possible in the allotted time. Whenever you repeat this workout you should strive to complete more reps than last time.

Timed repetitions

Simply set yourself the goal of a certain number of reps and try to complete it in as short a time as possible, e.g. 300 swings, 500 swings or even 1,000 swings. Whenever you repeat this workout you should strive to do it quicker than before.

Descending repetition pyramid

The sets in this workout get shorter as you get more tired - this means you can keep the intensity high from start to finish. Simply perform a high-rep set of swings, for example 20 reps, rest a few seconds and then repeat, but perform one less rep. Continue knocking off a rep per set until you get down to one. Perform this workout against the clock and try to beat your best time by swinging faster and resting less.

Hammer and callisthenic combinations

Alternate a set of hammer swings with a set of free-standing bodyweight exercises such as squats or lunges - this method ensures that the lower body gets a good workout along with the upper body and is a great way of getting a lot done in a short time.

Rocks, Breeze Blocks, Barrels and Logs

A 10kg (22 lb) medicine ball costs, at the time of writing, around £100. While medicine balls *are* versatile, that's a lot of money to tie up in a single piece of exercise equipment. You can replicate many medicine ball exercises using sandbags as detailed earlier, or using objects that you find lying around your training area. Rocks, stones and logs are great alternatives if you don't have access to weights. This form of training is often referred to as odd object lifting. Odd objects can be lifted and thrown just like a medicine ball, or used in place of barbells and dumbbells to replicate many strength-training exercises including dead lifts, thrusters and bent-over rows.

Old beer and water barrels are also effective (and often free) training tools. Filled with water or sand, they can be lifted, dragged and thrown to develop your endurance, strength or power. As when using a sandbag, the contents will move around as you exercise, which increases the demand placed on your core and joint stabilizing muscles.

Odd objects generally feel much heavier than the equivalent barbell or dumbbell. They tend to be more awkward to handle and, as such, their weight is relatively

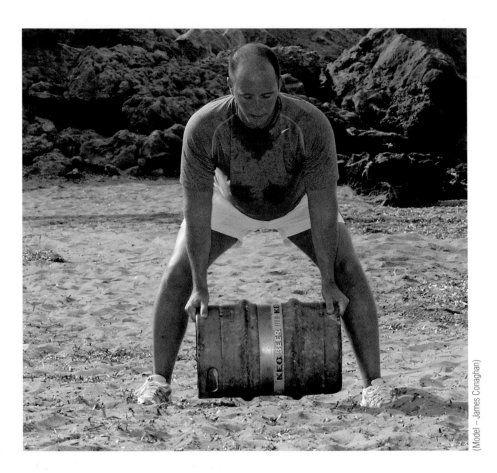

Barrels, rocks and ammo boxes are all viable workout tools.

(Model – James Conaghan)

unimportant when compared to how hard they make you work. It's easy to quantify the weight of a beer or water barrel as a litre of water weighs 1 kg (a little over 2 lb). However rocks and logs often feel heavier than they really are. Rather than worry about how heavy your odd object is, just work as hard as you can and try to work even harder next time. Remember, your body doesn't know if you are lifting a machine-calibrated Olympic barbell or a piece of rubble – it just knows it is heavy, and will get stronger accordingly.

Suspension Training Equipment

There are a number of manufacturers making suspension training equipment. A suspension trainer is an adjustable webbing strap with handles that is attached to an overhead anchor point that can then be used for the performance of a wide range of bodyweight exercises. The American military have adopted suspension training as one of their primary conditioning tools for soldiers on deployment. Suspension trainers are portable, lightweight and very versatile. They can turn regular body-weight exercises into very challenging movements and also allow you to perform some unique exercises that are otherwise impossible.

If you would like to try this form of exercise but you don't want to buy a suspension trainer, you can make one using adjustable haulage straps (the ones with ratchet tension adjusters), a couple of handles from a cable crossover machine and some climbing webbing loops. All in all you should be able to make one for about £50.00 or less.

Suspension training cannot replace lifting heavy weights, essential for developing real-world strength. However, it is very effective for improving muscular endurance, inter-joint and muscle coordination and also core and joint stability. Is it essential to your training? No, but it is a nice addition and can be considered a fair alternative if you don't have access to weights.

Resistance Bands

Resistance bands are a veritable gym in a bag! Cheap, highly portable and very versatile, a good set of resistance bands can replace an array of free weight exercises. That is not to say you should use resistance bands *instead of* free weights, but that you may wish to supplement your free weight training with some resistance band work.

Bands are ideal when you are training 'away from home' but don't want to be limited to bodyweight exercises. Many bands are adjustable, can be combined to alter the resistance and often come supplied with door anchors so that you can simulate virtually every free weight and machine strength-training exercise.

On the downside, resistance bands do not have the same 'feel' as free weights and the strength curve is completely reversed. Where a free weight tends to get easier as you approach lockout, the same exercise performed with a resistance band gets harder. This means that strength developed with resistance bands tends to be confined to the outer range of movement of any exercise you perform. That said, exercises such as band pull-aparts and the archer's pull are among the best postural upper back exercises available, irrespective of the equipment you choose to use.

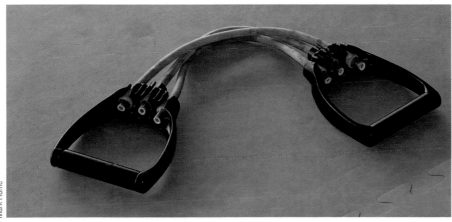

Mark Hume

Resistance bands – a viable if occasional alternative to free weights.

Weighted Vests

Soldiers on patrol normally wear some form of body armour as well as carrying ammo and essential supplies in a specially designed chest harness called webbing. Unlike kit in a rucksack, the weight is kept very close to your body, which means that the load is kept over your base of support and your balance is not drastically affected. Marines, for example, perform all of their commando fitness tests carrying 10 kg (22 lb) in their webbing. The civilian equivalent of body armour and/or webbing is the weighted vest.

Weighing between 4.5 and 36 kg (10 and 80 lb), most models of weighted vests are adjustable and come supplied with a number of metal ingots that can be removed or added to the vest to adjust your workload. A light weighted vest will make exercises such as press-ups and squats a little more challenging, whereas a heavy weighted vest can be used to develop real strength. Weighted vests are not recommended for running – at least, not by me. Running places enough impactful force through your body and adding even more is likely to result in injury. However, walking while wearing a weighted vest is a different matter altogether. Yomping long distances while carrying 18 kg (40 lb) plus of weight is a very effective cardiovascular workout and a supreme calorie burner. It strengthens your legs, hips and back and makes non-weighted activities much easier by comparison.

Weighted vests can be expensive but a good vest is a long-term investment that will last years. When choosing a vest, make sure you buy one you will 'grow into' in terms of loading capacity. A lighter vest may be cheaper but, once you have improved your fitness to the extent that you need a heavier vest, you'll have to buy a heavier one anyway. Buy the heaviest vest you can afford but only load it with the amount of weight you can carry comfortably. I suggest starting with around 10% of your bodyweight and adding half a kilo (a pound) every week or two. Be aware that a weighted vest can make you a little bit cumbersome – especially the first few times you use it. Stay on flat surfaces initially and progress to more challenging terrain as you get used to wearing your vest.

Weighted vests make even the easiest bodyweight exercise more challenging.

Vests are available in a number of styles but the main differences are the length of the body and the method by which the vest is fastened. Short vests keep your midsection free, which makes breathing easier but also limits carrying capacity. Longer vests allow you to carry more weight but also reduce movement at your spine, so they are better suited to walking and less suited to exercises that require mobility and ease of movement. Some vests use buckles and straps while others rely on Velcro fastenings. Both work well, but Velcro has a finite lifespan

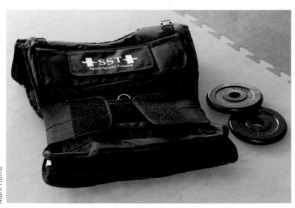

Mark Hume

after which it tends to gradually lose its adherence. Elastic also degrades and loses its spring, although it does allow for a more forgiving fit.

The main point to consider when buying a weighted vest is comfort. You might end up wearing your vest for a couple of hours during a yomp so it is essential that it doesn't rub, bounce, jiggle or otherwise make you wish you'd never bought the darn thing!

On a personal note, I have a long-bodied weighted vest with a maximum carrying capacity of 18 kg (40 lb). It is adjustable at the shoulders and waist. It's a few years old now and the degraded elastic and Velcro waist strap is almost ineffectual so I have to wrap an old leather belt around it to hold it in place. It isn't pretty, but it works.

If you prefer, instead of buying a weighted vest, you can simply load up a backpack with sandbags or weight plates wrapped in towels. This option is fine if you are just yomping along, but as soon as you try to run or perform any bodyweight exercises you will probably find the backpack moves all over the place. If it's comfort and a snug fit you are after, a weighted vest is best.

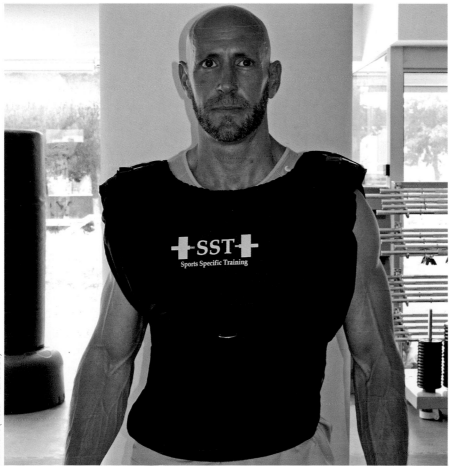

Mark Hume (Model – Patrick Dale)

A weighted vest looks and feels much like body armour!

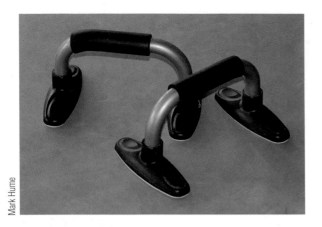

A firm forces favourite, press-up bars make the humble press-up much more demanding.

Press-up Bars

Whenever I went away on deployment, I could always guarantee that one of my fellow Marines would have remembered to pack his press-up bars. The military's love of press-ups is well documented and, consequently, anything that makes press-ups more challenging and therefore more effective is going to be well received by squaddies and bootnecks alike! Press-up bars make this prince of upper body exercises more demanding by allowing you to work your muscles through a greater than normal range of movement. Normally, when performing press-ups, you can only lower your chest to the floor, but press-up bars effectively lower the floor and provide you with more space to move. This increased range of movement means that your muscles must work harder. Combine press-up bars with a weighted vest or backpack and you have a chest exercise to rival the mighty bench press!

Dress for Success

Most soldiers have a myriad uniforms that must be worn according to the task of the day. As a Marine, I had uniforms for daily wear, a uniform for desert operations, one for jungle operations, my best parade blues and a second-best green parade uniform, arctic overalls and a dry suit for amphibious operations. The point of this list is not to tell you that I had more outfits than a well-dressed Action Man, but to illustrate that I always had the right clothing and equipment for the job in hand. You should be no different.

Exercise clothing is a personal choice. Some people like to work out in figure-hugging Lycra while others prefer loose-fitting cotton. Irrespective of your preferences, like any well-equipped soldier, your clothing should match the demands of your training. If you are comfortable, you are more likely to be able to exercise to the best of your ability. Poorly fitting exercise clothing can mean the difference between a great workout and knocking off early. Here is your ground-up guide to exercise clothing.

Shoes and Socks

Choosing a pair of exercise shoes can seem like a daunting prospect and, often, an expensive one. The shoe market is very competitive and each shoe manufacturer uses pseudo-scientific information to try to convince you that you *must* buy their ultra-light, super-supportive, gait-controlling foot-chariot. The truth is that most sports shoes are very similar, and only last a few months before the touted shock-absorbing and gait-controlling properties begin to break down; and the more engineered a shoe is, the less work your foot muscles are required to do, so the weaker and more reliant on these super-shoes your feet become – talk about a vicious circle!

Running shoes

Unless you are a specialist runner putting in 80 km (50 miles) or more a week you really don't need anything much more than a basic, firm but stable running shoe. Remember that the more supportive the shoe is, the weaker your feet will become so, unless you have a medically diagnosed gait anomaly, you probably don't need those £150 anti-pronation, feather-weight racing flats that skinny runner guy in the shop is trying to sell you. Running only makes up a small percentage of your weekly training programme, so don't feel obliged to blow your budget on specialist running shoes.

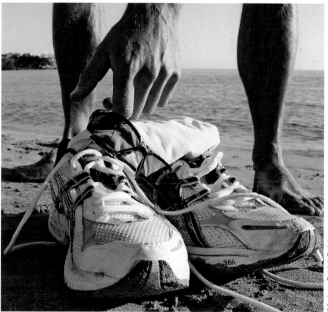

(Mode – Patrick Dale)

Make sure you have the right shoes for the job.

Gym shoes

A separate pair of shoes for gym training is not essential, but you may find it beneficial to keep one pair of shoes for your outdoor activities and another pair for indoors. This means that if your shoes get wet and muddy, you won't end up defiling your gym space and losing favour with your local gym manager or, if you train at home, your significant other! Because you won't be pounding the pavement in your gym shoes, these can be less cushioned and flatter in the heel than your running shoes. This lower profile can be quite advantageous when you are performing strength-training exercises as it means you tend to wobble less – very important when performing ground-based exercises such as squats or standing presses. Thick-soled shoes tend to compress, especially when you are performing squats, lunges or any other standing exercise. This makes the exercise more difficult to perform and also increases the wear and tear on your probably expensive running shoes. Low-tech is best for gym shoes.

Yomping shoes

There is nothing to stop you yomping in your running shoes but, as I hope you will be venturing off-road and into the wilds, you will be better served by wearing walking shoes or boots. Boots offer greater ankle support while shoes tend to be lighter, so

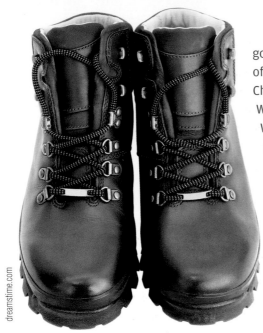

dreamstime.com

A soldier's boots can be his best friend or worst enemy, depending on their fit!

go with whatever suits you best. Shoes and boots are made of a variety of materials – both man-made and natural. Choose a material that is breathable but also water resistant. Waxed leather or Gore-tex-lined nylon is my preference. Wellington boots are not suitable for yomping! Before you set off on your first yomp, make sure you have spent a few days walking around your home and local area breaking in your boots and checking for hotspots. Blisters can reduce even the hardest soldier to his knees and are best avoided. For an authentic military yomping experience, you could always go down to your local Army and Navy surplus store and buy some genuine combat boots. Once they are broken in, you'll probably find that you never need another pair again, as they are the ultimate in hard-wearing footwear.

Socks

When choosing socks, stick with ones with no obvious seams that may rub and cause blisters. They should fit well and not move around on your feet, but also not be so tight that they cut into your ankles. You can spend £20 a pair on technical running socks or £2 a pair on regular cotton socks. All that matters is your comfort – financial as well as physical. Replace your socks if they begin to wear, get threadbare or lose their elasticity.

Socks for yomping must fit especially well as you could be in them for several hours at a time. Your yomp will be more enjoyable if your socks have padded heels and forefeet. Personally, I think the best walking socks are the standard military issue woollen sock in olive green. I've got a few pairs that are over ten years old and going strong while other, more 'technically advanced' and expensive socks have failed to last a single season.

Clothing
Underwear

As far as underwear goes, your most comfortable undergarments might be OK when strolling around the supermarket on a Friday evening, but could turn into an organ-constricting torture device when you exercise. Even worse, your civvie undergarments might not actually provide you with the support you need while working out. It's worth buying good-quality sports underwear that will hold your bits and pieces in place. Both men and women need to ensure they are well supported during exercise, as unfettered dangly bits are not just uncomfortable but can also lead to injury.

Military Fitness

Shorts and trousers

Whatever your preference for leg coverings, it's important that they aren't restrictive. In the grand scheme of things, it's up to you whether you wear long trousers or shorts for your running and workouts, but it is essential that you can move freely and you don't get cold or overheated. For yomping, a sturdy pair of cargo trousers or shorts will be useful so you have pockets in which you can safely transport your car keys, wallet, and mobile phone and maybe even a map, compass and energy gel.

Tops

I prefer to wear a vest or T-shirt when I exercise, but I live in Cyprus so cold weather is seldom an issue for me. If you live in colder climes you may need to wear more than just a lightweight top for your exercise sessions. It is important that you can 'vent' as your body temperature increases, so choose tops that have large zips or wear a couple of thin layers so that you can avoid getting overheated. Exercise is hard enough without having to contend with hyperthermia and dehydration! Many modern technical sports tops are made of wicking material which allows moisture, specifically sweat, to be drawn away from your skin for easy evaporation. This means you won't end up weighed down by a sweat-soaked T-shirt. Wicking tops cost more than a basic cotton T-shirt but may be a good investment if, like me, you sweat like the proverbial pig!

Outerwear

Inclement weather is one of life's unavoidable annoyances. If you put your training on hold every time the weather is less than ideal, you could find yourself only exercising for a few months a year. As we used to say in the Royal Marines: 'If it isn't raining, it isn't training!' Rather than avoiding poor weather, you can equip yourself so that you can exercise *irrespective* of the elements. A lightweight Gore-tex rain suit can make running in a torrential downpour much more tolerable. Fleece tops and thermal leggings can stop cold from being your enemy. Hats and gloves will keep your extremities dry and warm. 'Any fool can be cold and wet' is something of a mantra in military basic training and the trick is not to be that fool. A peaked hat can also be useful for keeping the sun out your eyes and off your head. Hats can help keep your unruly, long civilian hair in place or, if you are a baldy like me, stop you getting a sun-burnt scalp. I also find that a baseball hat or similar keeps sweat out of my eyes and is much more socially acceptable than the 80s alternative – the towelling sweat band.

Reflective clothing

If you intend to work out at night, you really should consider wearing some high visibility (hi-viz) clothing. This could be a bright, reflective tabard worn over your regular training clothing, or one of those putrid luminous green training tops favoured by marathon runners. Whatever you choose, it's better to be seen than to get hit by a motorist. Think of it as reverse camouflage. Combine your new, day-glo wardrobe with a head-torch for the ultimate in hi-viz chic!

Supplementary Kit

There's no denying that soldiers like kit. Anything that will make their lives a little bit easier in the field or save some valuable time that can then be spent sleeping or eating is very highly prized. If something is particularly useful, it is likely to be labelled as being 'Gucci'. For example, a pair of non-issue lightweight Gore-tex lined combat boots is considered very 'Gucci' despite not coming from an Italian fashion house! There are a number of 'Gucci' pieces of training equipment that, while not being really essential, can help make your training experience all the more enjoyable.

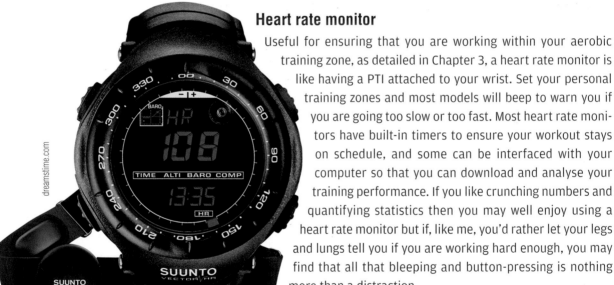

Heart rate monitor

Useful for ensuring that you are working within your aerobic training zone, as detailed in Chapter 3, a heart rate monitor is like having a PTI attached to your wrist. Set your personal training zones and most models will beep to warn you if you are going too slow or too fast. Most heart rate monitors have built-in timers to ensure your workout stays on schedule, and some can be interfaced with your computer so that you can download and analyse your training performance. If you like crunching numbers and quantifying statistics then you may well enjoy using a heart rate monitor but if, like me, you'd rather let your legs and lungs tell you if you are working hard enough, you may find that all that bleeping and button-pressing is nothing more than a distraction.

Technology can help you measure the intensity of your workout.

Feeding belt

Most of your workouts are pretty short, so it's unlikely you will need to take on lots of fluid or carbohydrate while you are exercising. The most notable exception to this is the weekly yomp. You have plenty of fat on your frame to fuel you for prolonged periods of exercise but 'fat must be burnt in a carbohydrate flame' and once you run low on stored carbohydrate, called muscle glycogen, you can be left feeling pretty weak and feeble. Marathon runners call this turn of events 'hitting the wall', while cyclists call it 'bonking' (stop sniggering at the back). You can prevent excessive glycogen depletion by taking on carbohydrates during your yomp and one of the easiest ways to do this is through sports drinks. Nutrition is covered in the next chapter but, needless to say, the more conveniently located your sports drink, the more likely you are to use it as a preventative measure as opposed to only when you need to – by which time it's probably too late. Feeding belts are usually made of neoprene, the same stuff as wetsuits, and have sufficient pockets to hold a couple of drinks bottles, some energy bars or gels, your MP3 player and your phone. This saves having to stick energy gels down your shorts – neither hygienic nor a good look.

MP3 player

Music has been proved to raise your psychological arousal levels and help motivate you towards a better workout. Although some exercisers find music distracting, for others it makes the difference between a ho-hum training session and giving it your all. It's really a case of finding what music has the most profound effect on your energy levels. For me, it's old-school rock like AC/DC, Iron Maiden, Deep Purple and other music that my parents generally classed as 'an awful noise'. Sometimes I like music in the background and at other times I want it loud and right in my ears. This means that, as often as I use my MP3 player with headphones, I also use it connected to an external loudspeaker. Experiment with music – it might be the missing piece you need to ramp up your exercise intensity. Please remember, however, that being able to hear can provide you with an effective early warning of impending danger. Do not use your MP3 player when out running or cycling, or at any other time when doing so increases your risk of accident or injury.

Sunglasses

Exercising in bright sunshine makes you squint. Squinting causes your facial muscles to tense up and, if left unchecked, this can lead to wrinkles. More importantly, tense facial muscles often result in tense neck muscles and tense neck muscles cause your shoulders to hunch up. Once this happens, your movements are likely to become much less economical and relaxed, which can lead to premature fatigue and a whole lot of neck and shoulder pain. Wearing sunglasses might seem over the top but anything that makes the whole exercise experience more comfortable is a worthwhile consideration. Sports sunglasses are light and cheap and protect your eyes from harmful ultraviolet radiation. Also, nothing stops a workout like grit in your eye and sunglasses can help you avoid this.

Sunscreen

Not so many years ago, sunscreens were thick, greasy and pore-clogging and required very frequent application. Modern sunscreens are lightweight and don't need to be layered on so thickly that your skin can't breathe. If you exercise outdoors during the heat of the summer, a sunscreen is a worthwhile addition to your training kit. If you are pale skinned or otherwise unused to prolonged sun exposure, a good dose of midday sun can leave you red and sore. This is especially likely during your longer yomps. *Some* sun exposure is very good for you and helps with, among other things, vitamin D production, but too much sun can do you harm. One of the main problems with sunburn is that you often don't realize you are burnt until after it has happened and by then the damage is done. An ounce of prevention is worth a pound of cure, so make like an Australian out-backer and slip, slop, slap – that's slip on a shirt, slop on the sunscreen and slap on a hat.

Backpack

When yomping, you will need something in which to carry your waterproofs, first aid kit and trail food and the most comfortable way to do it is in a backpack. Backpacks are available in a variety of sizes which are normally described in terms of litres of capacity. A small 'day pack' will usually be between 15 and 25 litres in size and should be ample for a few hours out in the wilds of your local park. If you are intending to go further afield, a larger pack may be necessary, so look for sizes in the 30 to 40 litre range. If in doubt, buy a bigger pack rather than a smaller one as you can always partially fill a big pack but if you have too much kit to fit in a small pack, you will have to spend more money and buy another.

Your backpack – part workout accessory, part luggage solution; essential for yomps.

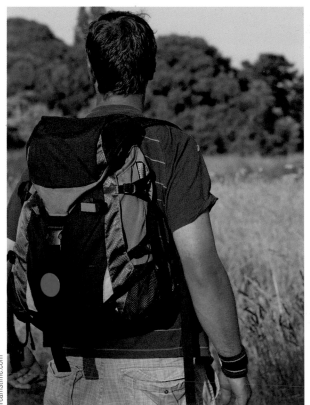

dreamstime.com

Another consideration when selecting a backpack is the storage area arrangement. Some packs consist of a single storage compartment while others have multiple compartments and pockets so that you can spread your gear around and have easy access. Another thing to consider is how the pack fits you. A badly fitting backpack can make a yomp a miserable experience. Narrow straps cut into your shoulders, and if the pack does not fit snugly to your body you may find it moves around and rubs your skin. In the Marines this is called Bergen rash and, while it's common in Marine recruits, there is no reason you should suffer such an inconvenience! A waist belt can help keep the back firmly in place and also takes some of the weight off your shoulders. A good pack should last for years, so think of this purchase as a long-term investment.

Your kitbag is packed so now let's move on to most soldiers' favourite subject – food!

CHAPTER SEVEN

Nutrition

Fuelling the big, green military fitness machine!

The focal point of any armed forces establishment is not the gym or the parade square but where the men and women eat. The galley in naval terms, called the cookhouse by the Army, this is where the soldiers, sailors and airmen come to replenish their energy supplies as well as enjoy some down-time with friends and workmates.

It's always been said that an army marches on its belly. Food, or more accurately the lack of it, has been responsible for some of the greatest military defeats throughout the ages. Starve your enemy, break their supply lines and it's normally not too long before you see the white flag of surrender flying in the wind.

Like any army, ancient or modern, you need a good supply of high-quality nutrients to keep your body's systems functioning properly. Consider a Formula One racing car: If you put low-grade fuel in the tank, chances are that the car will run badly, if at all, and be much more prone to mechanical breakdown. Your body is a far more complex piece of equipment than any car and requires optimum fuelling for smooth running. The best programme, the most intense workouts, the most diligent attention to following the exercise principles, will all be for nothing if you do not fuel your body properly. Of course, you will make *some* progress - your body's adaptation to exercise is based on the age-old survival mechanisms that are hard-wired into your genes. But will you see the results you deserve if you are training hard but eating badly? Not bloomin' likely!

Does this mean that you need to learn the complete A to Z of nutrition, measure everything you eat and drink and buy expensive food supplements? Thankfully not. Getting your nutritional intake right is a relatively simple process. That's not to say nutrition is a simple subject - far from it. But using the car analogy again, you don't need to know everything about the petrochemical industry to know that you shouldn't put diesel in a Formula One car. It's not rocket science, just common sense.

In this chapter you'll find a broad and simple overview of the main nutrient groups so you can better understand what they do, where they come from and how much you need. Don't worry - there won't be a test at the end and you won't need to weigh your food or start buying any weird and exotic ingredients. Like the exercise programme in this book, your nutritional brief is stripped down, simple, practical and nonsense-free!

Macronutrients

Macro means big. The macronutrients make up the majority of your food intake. They provide energy for activity and the building blocks of the cells that make up your body. There are three macronutrient groups – proteins, carbohydrates and fats.

Proteins

Protein is a vital nutrient that makes up a large amount of your body's tissues including your hair, skin, nails and bones and, of course, your muscles. The word protein is derived from the Greek word *proto* (primary or first), but protein is actually made up from smaller units called amino acids. Amino acids can be thought of as the protein alphabet although, unlike letters in the English alphabet, there are only 20 amino acids.

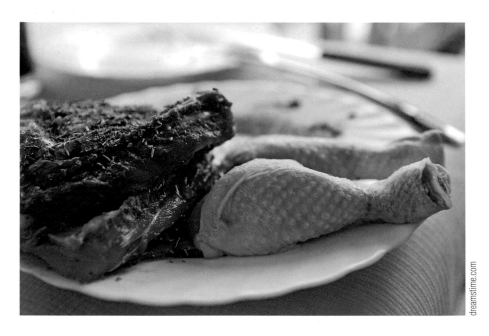

Protein foods such as beef and chicken provide essential amino acids.

Amino acids are classified as essential or non-essential. There are eight or nine essential amino acids that must be present in your diet. Why eight or nine? Some controversy surrounds the amino acid histidine (sometimes called histamine) and whether it is essential for adults or just children. The remaining (whether eleven or twelve) non-essential amino acids are synthesized by your liver, provided that the essential amino acids are present in your diet.

When you eat a protein food, for example chicken, your body breaks down the food into its constituent amino acids and uses them for whatever purpose is required at the time. This includes growth and repair of muscle tissue after exercise, the manufacture of hormones such as insulin and growth hormone, and even as a source of energy – although this only happens if there is no other fuel available.

Complete and incomplete proteins

Foods that contain adequate amounts of all the essential amino acids are classed as 'complete'. Complete proteins include eggs, meat, fish, dairy produce, poultry, soya and quinoa. A diet rich in these foods means that you have all the amino acids necessary to synthesize the non-essential amino acids.

Many plants contain a variety of amino acids but are often deficient in some of the essentials and are therefore classed as 'incomplete' proteins. Because they are lacking one or more of the essential amino acids, most plant foods are considered to be carbohydrates rather than proteins. Examples include vegetables, seeds, nuts, beans and grains.

Complementary proteins

Like pieces of a jigsaw, you can slot incomplete proteins together to make a fully fledged protein. It's simply a matter of making sure that, between them, the incomplete proteins supply all of the essential amino acids in sufficient amounts. A protein made up in this way is called a complementary protein and provides a convenient way to obtain adequate dietary protein without having to eat any actual protein foods. There are a number of food combinations you can use to form a complementary protein (see below).

Grains and pulses
Vegetables and nuts
Vegetables and seeds
Grains and dairy
Nuts and seeds
Nuts and pulses
Seeds and pulses

With a little culinary imagination it is possible to turn any of the incomplete proteins listed into a healthy source of complete protein – or, at the least, put some peanut butter on your toast or some nuts in your vegetable stir-fry!

Rating protein

Protein foods are rated in terms of quality, using a number of different scales. The various scales evaluate the digestibility of a protein and the availability of essential amino acids. The greater the amount of the consumed protein that can be utilized by your body, the higher the score will be. Most proteins of animal origin, such as eggs, meat and fish, and also soya, score very highly whereas incomplete proteins such as beans score much lower.

The best-known scale for protein quality is the Biological Value Scale (BV for short); other scales include Net Protein Utilization (NPU), Protein Efficiency Ratio (PER) and the Protein Digestibility Corrected Amino Acid Score (PDCAAS). Each rating method is slightly different and uses a variety of criteria for scoring a protein, hence the variations in the chart below.

Protein Source	Rating Method			
	BV	NPU	PER	PDCAAS
Whey protein	104	92	3.6	1.0
Whole egg	100	94	3.8	1.0
Beef	80	73	2.0	0.92
Casein (milk)	77	76	2.9	1.0
Soy	74	61	2.1	0.99
Rice	59	57	2.0	0.26
Beans	49	39	1.4	0.68

Protein recommendations and requirements

Protein recommendations vary from nutritional expert to nutritional expert, but the general consensus of opinion is that you need around 1.6 to 2.0 g per kg of body-weight per day. Does this mean that you need to weigh and measure your food to ensure you are getting enough protein? Not really – simply make sure that each meal that you consume includes a portion of good-quality protein and you'll be well on your way to making sure you get enough of this vital nutrient.

However, it's not just the *quantity* of the protein you should consider but the actual food *quality* as well. As the old adage goes, 'If you put junk in, you'll get junk out', so it pays to try to consume the best-quality protein foods you can. Lean organic meats and poultry, free-range eggs, organic milk and raw nuts are all good sources of protein that will provide amino acids and other essential nutrients.

Not-so-good protein choices include burgers, sausages, meat pies, UHT dairy, roasted nuts, non-organic pulses, re-formed meats such as luncheon meat and battery-farmed eggs. Re-formed and processed meats often contain as little as 6% actual meat (a figure allowable by law!), and much of their weight consists of water and fillers such as wheat, sugar and bone meal. Corned beef is often referred to as corned dog in military circles. While I doubt there is any actual dog in a can of corned beef, you can be assured that at least some of the contents are derived from parts of the animal you wouldn't eat if given the choice!

Carbohydrates

Carbohydrates are plant foods that are made up from sugar molecules called saccharides. Saccharides are found singly, in pairs and in complicated chains. The structure of a carbohydrate dictates how it is categorized. Carbohydrates provide 4 calories per gram (or around 16.8 kilojoules) and are the preferred source of energy for your brain and for higher-intensity activities such as weightlifting and sprinting. In short – the more active you are, the greater your need for a plentiful supply of carbohydrates.

Simple carbohydrates

Simple carbohydrates can be found in two forms – monosaccharides and disaccharides. Monosaccharides consist of single saccharide molecules, whereas disaccharides are pairs of molecules joined together. Simple carbohydrates are often referred to as 'sugars', which carries negative connotations for some people, with the possible implication that all simple carbohydrates are bad for you. While sugar is a simple carbohydrate – a disaccharide called sucrose to be precise – not all simple carbohydrates are sugars! Most fruit is also a simple carbohydrate and everyone knows just how good fruit is for you. In addition to fruit and fruit derivatives such as juices and dried fruit, simple carbohydrates are also commonly found in confectionery, sports drinks, dairy products and energy bars.

There are three primary monosaccharides – glucose, fructose and galactose, and three primary disaccharides – sucrose (glucose and fructose), lactose (glucose and galactose) and maltose (glucose bonded to glucose).

Monosaccharides – single molecules or 'units' of sugar

Glucose

Fructose

Galactose

Disaccharides – two molecules or 'units' of sugar joined together e.g.

Sucrose = glucose + fructose

Lactose = glucose + galactose

Maltose = glucose + glucose

Complex carbohydrates

Complex carbohydrates are made from multiple chains of saccharide molecules called polysaccharides – poly meaning many. Polysaccharides are also called starches. Starches make up the greatest percentage of most people's food intake and can be found in bread, rice, pasta, vegetables and grain-based foods.

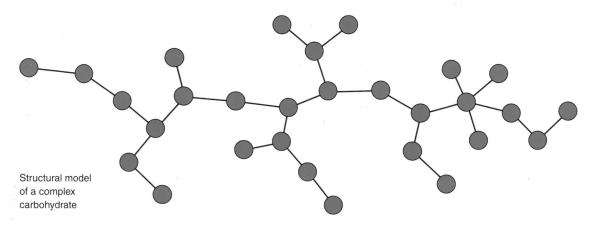

Structural model of a complex carbohydrate

The fate of dietary carbohydrate

Whatever type of carbohydrate you consume, all carbohydrate is broken down by digestive enzymes called pancreatic and salivary amylase and turned into glucose. Your body has a number of different uses for glucose.

Once digested, glucose enters your bloodstream and stimulates your pancreas to release the hormone insulin. Insulin acts like a key to unlock your cells and allows the glucose to enter various tissues. Glucose is stored for later use in the form of glycogen, used for fuel or, if there is an excess, converted to fat. A small amount of glucose also remains in your blood and is the primary fuel for your brain.

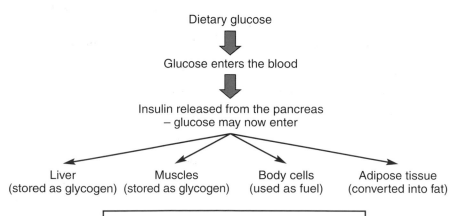

The fate of dietary carbohydrates

Glycogen is locked into your liver or muscles. Liver glycogen provides a reservoir of glucose for your brain, whereas muscle glycogen provides energy for contractions of the muscles in which it is stored.

Refined and unrefined carbohydrates

Both simple and complex forms of carbohydrate can be further classified according to the degree of processing or refinement that they have undergone. As a general rule, the more refined a product is the less fibre and fewer vitamins and minerals it will contain, and therefore the less healthy it becomes. While it is unrealistic to suggest that you should eliminate all simple refined carbohydrates from your diet, it is worth noting that, in general, refined carbohydrates are largely stripped of all important nutrients and are less healthful than their unrefined counterparts.

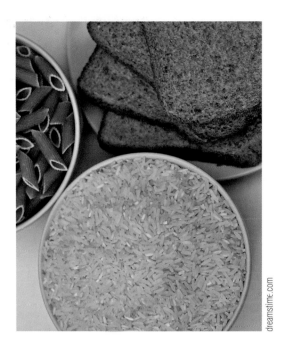

dreamstime.com

Bread, rice and pasta are all sources of complex carbohydrates.

Refined Simple Carbohydrates	Refined Complex Carbohydrates
• Sweets	• White bread
• Desserts	• White pasta
• Confectionery	• White rice
• Sugar	• Rice cakes
• Pasteurized/concentrated fruit juice	• Pastries
• Soda/soft drinks	• Cakes
	• Carbohydrate content of processed food
Unrefined Simple Carbohydrates	**Unrefined Complex Carbohydrates**
• Fresh fruit	• Wholegrain bread
• Non-pasteurized/concentrated fruit juice	• Wholemeal pasta
• Dried fruit	• Vegetables
	• Potatoes
	• Pulses
	• Wholegrain cereals e.g. oats, rye, spelt

The glycaemic index

Not all carbohydrates have been created equal and some sources of carbs are definitely healthier than others in terms of nutritional density. It's easy enough to select which carbohydrates contain the least amount of refined sugars and greatest number of micronutrients, but there is yet another way by which carbohydrates are classified.

The glycaemic index is a scoring system that rates carbohydrates according to the speed at which they are digested and converted into blood glucose. The glycaemic index uses a 1-100 scale. Fast-acting carbohydrates score very highly, while slower-acting carbohydrates get more moderate scores. The glycaemic index gives you a good indication of which carbohydrates to eat when. There are numerous interpretations of what constitutes a low, moderate or high glycaemic index but the following chart is fairly representative of the accepted norms.

- **High Glycaemic Index – 60 to 100**

- **Moderate Glycaemic Index – 40 to 60**

- **Low Glycaemic Index – Below 40**

High glycaemic foods such as sugary cereals, refined grain products and confectionery are quickly digested and converted to usable glucose. This makes them ideal if you need a quick burst of energy during or just before a workout, or want to refuel as fast as possible after a workout.

Low glycaemic index foods such as beans, apples, most dairy and porridge oats take longer to digest and will release their energy more slowly. This means that you tend to feel fuller for longer after eating low glycaemic index carbohydrates and experience more stable energy levels throughout the day as a result.

As with all of your food choices, try to select the most nutritionally dense form of carbohydrate that you can. Although all carbohydrates provide energy, they are by no means equal in terms of vitamin, mineral and fibre density. Given the choice between a fresh apple and a cookie, the apple should be your food of choice – most of the time anyway!

Fibre

Fibre is, in fact, part of the carbohydrate group (it's actually a non-starch polysaccharide or NSP), but we'll look at it individually because of its particular characteristics. Found in the skin and flesh of plants, fibre is indigestible in the human gut, so is essentially calorie free. Despite this, or in fact because of this, fibre is a very important part of your diet.

Types of fibre

Fibre is classed as either soluble or insoluble – this refers to its interaction with water. Soluble fibre mixes with water and forms a gel-like substance, whereas insoluble fibre does not. Both forms of fibre provide a number of health benefits.

Benefits

Fibre delays the digestive process by remaining in your stomach for longer than other food items. This means that fibrous foods make you feel fuller for longer and also fuller, sooner. This is useful for weight management. By delaying gastric emptying, fibre also helps control blood glucose levels. Stable blood glucose levels mean less insulin production and therefore more stable energy levels and, as insulin suppresses fat burning, an increased use of fat for fuel.

By their nature, fibrous foods are generally more filling and take longer to eat than other food items. An apple and a cookie contain similar amounts of calories, but the fibrous content of apples means one or maybe two are all you want to eat in a single sitting. The same is not true of fibre-devoid cookies!

Fibre adds bulk to your stools to increase the transit time of waste material through your large intestine. This results in less digestive distress, less constipation, easier bowel movements, reduced incidence of diverticular disease and better digestive health generally. Fibre acts as an internal scrub to keep your digestive organs in good condition.

Soluble fibre absorbs a small amount of dietary fat, cholesterol and bile as it passes through your intestines. This can help lower serum triglyceride and cholesterol levels as well as reducing stomach wall damage caused by excess bile acid production.

Sources of fibre

As previously mentioned, fibre is found in plants. Soluble fibre comes from the fleshy parts of plants, for example beans, the flesh of apples and oranges, or the soft part of oats and other grains. Insoluble fibre is found in the tough husks of grains and the skins of fruits and vegetables, for example apple skins, wild rice and unrefined wheat products such as wholemeal bread.

The easiest way to ensure that you are getting enough fibre is to try to eat whole fruits, vegetables and unrefined grains at most meals. Most refined fruits, vegetables and grains are nearly devoid of fibre as it has been removed in the numerous stages of food preparation.

How much fibre do you need?

If you eat unrefined fruit, vegetables and grains with most meals you should have no problem hitting your optimum fibre intake of 35 g (1¼ oz) per day. If you think you are getting less than this, don't suddenly double your fibre intake overnight, as this

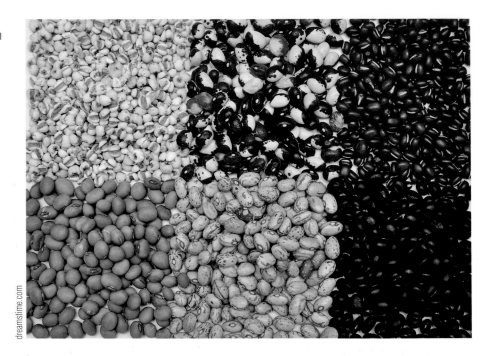

Vegetables, fruits, beans and grains all provide essential fibre in your diet.

dreamstime.com

can lead to abdominal bloating, discomfort, gas and constipation. Increase your fibre intake gradually over a few weeks until you reach the required amount. It is important to consume adequate water with your fibre as failure to do so can make your stools hard and uncomfortable to pass. We'll be discussing hydration later but for now, remember to consume around 2 litres (3½ pints) of water per day to keep your intestines functioning properly.

Fats

Fat is the most energy-dense food group and provides around 9 calories per gram. This high energy density is one of the primary reasons why many weight management plans focus on reducing fat intake. A relatively small decrease in fat intake will result in a significant decrease in calories consumed.

Fat is your primary source of energy during low-intensity aerobic activity. Right now, as you sit and read this book, you are using almost exclusively fat for fuel. As activity intensity levels increase, fat oxidation begins to decrease and carbohydrate-derived glucose oxidation increases until the point at which you are working anaerobically and your body switches almost exclusively to using carbohydrates for fuel. The phenomenon is responsible for the so-called 'fat-burning zone' that suggests that low-intensity exercise is the best tool for weight management. Is this actually the case? Like the high fat/low fat discussion, that's a subject for another book!

There are four main types of dietary fats – saturated, monounsaturated, polyunsaturated and trans fats. Each fat has a very specific chemical structure which dictates its role in your body.

Saturated fats

Often considered the 'bad boys' of dietary fats, saturated fats are composed of chains of carbon atoms that are packed or 'saturated' with hydrogen. This makes them, with the exception of palm oil and coconut oil, solid at room temperature. Saturated fats are chemically inert; they do not react very much to heat, light or oxygen and are ideal for cooking. Foods such as butter, animal produce, eggs and dairy contain large amounts of saturated fat.

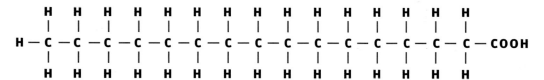

A model of the chemical structure of a saturated fat

Your body likes to use saturated fats for energy during aerobic activity, for storing for later use within your adipose tissue (fat cells), for protection of vital organs, for cell membrane integrity, and for the transport and storage of fat-soluble vitamins. They are also essential for protein utilization.

Monounsaturated fats

A monounsaturated fat is missing some hydrogen and, as a result, a double bond is formed in the carbon chain. The double bond causes a bend in the carbon chain and, in chemistry, shape dictates function. This means that a monounsaturated fat behaves differently from a saturated fat.

A model of the chemical structure of a monounsaturated fat

Monounsaturated fats are moderately reactive and more susceptible than saturated fats to changes caused by heat, light and oxygen. Liquid at room temperature, monounsaturated fats are linked to cardiovascular health and feature heavily in the olive oil-rich Mediterranean diet. Other sources of monounsaturated fats include nuts and nut-derived oils and butters, beef, avocados and numerous seeds.

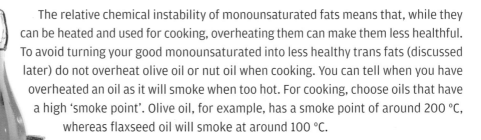

The relative chemical instability of monounsaturated fats means that, while they can be heated and used for cooking, overheating them can make them less healthful. To avoid turning your good monounsaturated into less healthy trans fats (discussed later) do not overheat olive oil or nut oil when cooking. You can tell when you have overheated an oil as it will smoke when too hot. For cooking, choose oils that have a high 'smoke point'. Olive oil, for example, has a smoke point of around 200 °C, whereas flaxseed oil will smoke at around 100 °C.

Polyunsaturated fats

Polyunsaturated fats contain two or more double bonds in their carbon chains. This characteristic makes them highly reactive when exposed to heat, light or oxygen. Examples of polyunsaturated fats include oily fish, sunflower seeds, sesame seeds, walnuts, soya beans and any oils subsequently extracted from these sources. The inherent reactivity seen in polyunsaturated fats means that exposing an otherwise healthy polyunsaturated fat to high temperatures is likely to result in the formation of trans fats. Polyunsaturated fats are not ideal oils for cooking; more stable saturated and monounsaturated fats are the better choice. Consume the majority of your polyunsaturated fats in a raw state to maximize their healthfulness.

Many polyunsaturated fats are considered essential for health, hence their common name 'essential fatty acids' (EFAs for short), and they can be subcategorized as omega 3 or omega 6 fatty acids. Omega, the final letter in the Greek alphabet, refers to the position in the chain at which the last double bend is located, i.e. three from the end or six from the end. These extremely healthful fats are responsible for a wide range of functions within your body, including the formation of cellular hormone-like substances called prostaglandins, the regulation of inflammation, mental function and development, and health of the skin, hair and immune system. Your granny may take cod liver oil to help 'lubricate her joints' but, in fact, cod liver oil is an effective anti-inflammatory agent and helps reduce joint pain rather than increasing lubrication!

Trans fats

Trans fats occur in nature and, when consumed in relatively small amounts, do not present any real problems for your health. However, many man-made foods and modern food preparation methods result in an abundance of trans fats being formed and consumed. Over-consumption of trans fats is strongly linked to immune system dysfunction, bone and tendon weakness, sterility, coronary heart disease, high cholesterol and triglyceride levels, inability to lactate, learning difficulties and low birth-weight babies.

Olive oil – a good source of monounsaturated fats

Military Fitness

Trans fats 'block' healthy mono and polyunsaturated fats from entering cells, resulting in impairment of cellular function which may lead to poor health.

Normal placement of hydrogen atoms
– as seen in a mono or polyunsaturated fat

Diagonal placement of hydrogen
atoms – as seen in a trans fat

You can minimize your consumption of trans fats by not overheating mono and polyunsaturated fats, cutting down on processed and takeaway foods, using saturated fats for high-temperature cooking and avoiding food products that contain hydrogenated vegetable oils. It is also a good idea to keep your mono and polyunsaturated oils in dark glass air-tight containers, buy extra-virgin cold-pressed oils and consider using butter instead of margarine as many margarine-type spreads contain hydrogenated vegetable oils. Check the label to be sure.

Fats – not as bad for us as we are often led to believe?

Many of the health problems associated with fats arise from the simple fact that they can make you fat. Being over-fat presents a much greater health risk than fats alone ever could. Your body needs a certain amount of fat for health and eliminating fat from your diet can lead to a host of medical problems. By being more 'fat aware' you can make sure you consume the fats that are best for you while avoiding those that can cause you harm.

Micronutrients

Micro means small, but that doesn't mean that this nutrient group is any less important than the macronutrients. It could even be said that the micronutrients are actually *more* important. There are two micronutrient groups – vitamins and minerals.

Vitamins

Vitamins come in two forms – water-soluble (vitamins B and C) and fat-soluble (vitamins A, D, E and K). Water-soluble vitamins cannot be stored in your body and must be consumed every day, whereas fat-soluble vitamins can be stored so they need only be consumed a few times a week. Both types of vitamins are essential to your health and wellbeing. In fact, the original definition of a vitamin was 'a substance that, if missing from the diet, will result in ill-health'. Vitamins were really only discovered at the beginning of the twentieth century and are named in order of their discovery. As nutritional science advances, so does our understanding of vitamins and the chemicals in our food. We now know which vitamin deficiencies are associated with which diseases. In case you were wondering, you obtain vitamins mainly from plants and also from animals that have eaten plants. Your intestinal tract can also synthesize some small amounts of essential vitamins.

What do vitamins do? They are the biological catalysts that are responsible for every chemical reaction in your body! Insufficient vitamins mean fewer, slower or non-existent reactions and, as per the definition earlier, ill-health is likely to be the result.

Scurvy, Limeys and Yanks

Back in the old days of the British Empire, British sailors could spend months or even years onboard one of His or Her Majesty's ships. On long voyages such as these, fruit and vegetables did not really feature in a sailor's diet as there was no way to refrigerate food and other methods of preservation such as salting, drying and pickling resulted in degradation of the vitamin content of food. Because of this general lack of the correct nutrients for long periods of time, British sailors often developed an immune system disease called scurvy. Sores, pustules and eye problems resulted in many sailors being unfit for duty, or even dying and ending up as fish food. To help treat scurvy, the Royal Navy ensured that all ships on long voyages were well stocked with limes as, although vitamin C had yet to be discovered, doctors had made the association between increased fruit intake and decreased scurvy outbreaks. From this point on, Americans nicknamed British sailors Limeys – a nickname that has subsequently been extended to all English people.

Minerals

Minerals are inorganic compounds that make up the soil in which our food grows. The plants absorb minerals and we eat the plants. It's the circle of life! Minerals can be classed as structural, as in the calcium in your bones, or homeostatic, for example sodium and its effect on fluid levels in your body. Minerals are only needed in very small amounts but they are as essential as vitamins for your wellbeing. For example, an iron deficiency will affect the oxygen-carrying ability of your blood and can result in a condition called anaemia. Lack of calcium can lead to osteoporosis and too much sodium can drive your blood pressure sky-high. These micronutrients are very powerful.

Getting What You Need

The best way to get all the micronutrients you require for good health is by eating real food. Eat a wide variety of plant and, if appropriate for you, animal foods and generally try to avoid overly processed foods devoid of good nutrition. In addition to the named vitamins and minerals that are present in your food, there are also tens of thousands of other known-to-be healthful chemicals in the fruit, vegetables, animal matter and grains you eat. There is no way even the most advanced nutritional supplement will contain all of these chemicals. If you so wish, you can use a multi-vitamin and mineral supplement to add to an already nutritionally sound diet, but don't try to prop up a bad diet with a couple of pills – it just won't work. (Supplements are dealt with further at the end of this chapter.)

Water and Hydration

Water is a calorie-free fluid that is essential for life. You can live quite a long time without food (depending on the size of your body fat stores) but only a few days without water. Water makes up around 70% of your total body mass and, to stop you getting dangerously dehydrated, your body uses thirst to tell you when to drink.

How Your Body Uses Water

Water acts as a suspension medium for all the chemicals in your body. Without water, these chemicals would have no way of mixing together or moving around your body. For example, plasma is the suspension medium for your various blood cells. No water? No way to circulate oxygen-carrying red blood cells, infection-fighting white blood cells or clotting platelets.

Your body uses water as a lubricant. Your joints, skin, eyes and digestive system function smoothly because of the presence of water. Like a car with no oil, your body would soon cease to function smoothly without water.

Water is also used to help detoxify your organs: water is flushed though your digestive system and kidneys so that toxins can be eliminated via your urine. Have you ever noticed how much more smelly and dark your urine is when you are dehydrated? That's the increased concentration of toxins you can smell. Staying well hydrated means that you are better able to flush these potentially harmful metabolic remnants out of your system.

Your body also uses water for temperature control. When you get too warm your body produces sweat, which subsequently evaporates and helps dissipate heat. You can lose a lot of water through sweating! Vigorous exhalations (panting) also result in water loss. The breath you can see on a cold day is, in fact, water vapour. It's still there when you exhale in warm weather – you just can't see it.

How Much Water do You Need?

Opinions vary, but consensus suggests that you need around 2 litres (3½ pints) of water per day plus a further half litre (just under a pint) per 30 minutes of exercise. Drinking more is not likely to cause you any harm as excesses will be eliminated.

Tea, coffee and juices, as well as fruit and vegetables, all contribute to your fluid intake as well, but as it's hard to estimate just how much water these sources provide, you should simply shoot for 2 litres (3½ pints) of water per day as a minimum. If you are getting thirsty, your body is telling you that you need to take some more water on board. Ignoring your thirst can actually desensitize you to the message your brain is sending and, although you might not feel thirsty, you may still be dehydrated. As a general rule, your urine output should be regular, copious and mostly clear and odour-free.

Sports Drinks

Sports drinks are designed to rehydrate you and also provide you with energy in the form of carbohydrates. Different sports drinks contain different amounts of carbohydrates and contents vary from 2 to 10 g per 100 ml. Sports drinks are great for long and gruelling workouts, but are merely a source of unwanted calories for most

Sports drinks may enhance your exercise performance.

general exercisers. Some 'light' sports drinks contain no carbohydrate but use artificial sweeteners, flavours and colours. These chemicals are often linked to health problems like attention deficit disorder (ADD), anxiety and hyperactivity and are generally best avoided. In the majority of cases, regular exercisers are best served by drinking plenty of plain water. If you find you are running low on energy during a workout of 60 minutes or less, the fault lies with your diet and not your choice of sports drink.

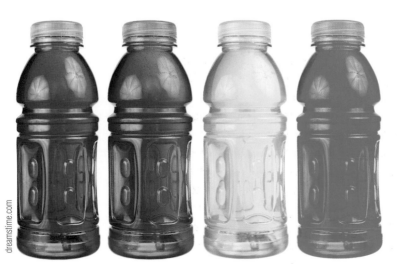

Military Fitness

Putting it all Together

The main thing to remember when designing your nutritional plan is that you should always eat for what you are about to do and what you have just done. By this I mean that, if you have a hard workout coming up, you need to ensure that you have eaten enough carbohydrate so you have sufficient fuel on board to power you through your workout. If you are, instead, about to sit at your desk all day, then you don't need as much carbohydrate, so protein and fats are more appropriate. In the hours after a workout, your muscles are like dried-out sponges and need a rapid supply of protein and carbohydrate to kick-start the recovery process. When you use the 'eat for what you are about to do and what you have just done' rule, deciding what food to eat and when is easy!

Meal Frequency

Most nutritional experts agree that smaller, more frequent meals are the best way to keep your blood glucose levels stable, avoid hunger and ensure that your muscles receive a steady supply of essential nutrients. *How* frequent depends on your personal preference and it's worth considering that three meals a day is considered high-frequency in some studies. Two large meals and two snacks is one option; three meals and two snacks is another. Some experts suggest that eating every three waking hours is ideal. The truth is that you have to find the eating schedule that fits seamlessly into your daily routine. The best diet in the world is useless if you can't actually stick to it!

Personally, I favour three meals and three snacks a day. I like eating, so frequent feedings are enjoyable for me. On the downside, it means that I have to carry food with me almost wherever I go and I spend the first part of every day getting my grub together when I'd much rather be getting an extra half-hour of sleep. More frequent feeding means you need to be well organized, but the trade-off is that you get to eat more often!

Pre-exercise feeding

Although your body has an abundant source of energy in the form of fat, you also need to keep your blood glucose levels stable, otherwise you may find you feel fatigued, nauseous, faint or weak part-way through your workout. Remember that fat is 'burnt in the flame of carbohydrate', which means that, despite fat being the most abundant source of energy in your body, you need carbs for fuel as well. Running out of muscle glycogen mid-workout results in a 'crash' in energy. This crash is technically called hypoglycaemia and describes a condition where your blood glucose levels drop too low and your brain starts to show the symptoms of being deprived of glucose. While not overly serious, hypoglycaemia may result in a substandard workout and may even mean that you have to break off your training early. Eating appropriately before exercise can ensure that you don't experience a blood glucose crash.

There are numerous opinions as to how best to feed your body prior to exercise. Some experts suggest a regular meal 2 hours prior to exercise while others believe that a fast-acting carbohydrate drink 15 minutes before your workout is ideal. Some experts suggest that you combine both of these methods. The most important thing to consider is that you avoid doing long and/or tough workouts if you are not adequately fuelled up! If you are an early morning trainer, this may mean you chug a sports drink as soon as you get out of bed to make sure you have plenty of fuel onboard to power you through your workout. If you train later in the day, you may want to have a carbohydrate-rich lunch so you are sufficiently energized for your workout. Experiment with a few approaches and see which method gives you the best results. We all respond differently to food and, while some people find they can comfortably exercise within an hour of eating, others may need 2–3 hours before they are ready to exercise.

Post-exercise feeding

After exercise, your body is primed to take up nutrients quickly to kick-start the repair and recovery process. Your muscles are like wrung-out sponges and will absorb nutrients at a much faster rate than usual. This is caused by a phenomenon called insulin sensitivity. Insulin is the hormone responsible for transporting glucose and amino acids into your cells and in the 15 minutes to 2-hour period after exercise, insulin sensitivity is at its most elevated. This means that most of the food you eat during this post-exercise window of opportunity is likely to be shunted into your liver and muscles.

You can make the most of your post-exercise insulin sensitivity and increase your workout recovery by making sure you consume fast-acting high-glycaemic carbohydrates and protein immediately after you finish your workout. This can be in the form of a specially designed post-exercise liquid meal or something as simple as a chicken sandwich on white bread. While a liquid meal will be digested more quickly, provided that you begin your post-exercise feed as soon as you can, real food is a very close second. Whatever you choose, make sure you are getting plenty of protein and carbohydrates, but go easy on the fat and fibre as these nutrients delay gastric emptying and consequently slow the release of nutrients into your blood.

Peri-exercise feeding

Peri-exercise feeding is a relatively new concept in sports nutrition and describes ingesting fuel before your workout ends to kick-start the recovery process even faster than would be possible if you were to rely on post-exercise feeding alone. Followers of peri-nutrition suggest that you should consume liquid protein and carbohydrates *during* your workout and not just at the end. Although this might be beneficial, non-stop exercise programmes such as the troop phyz workouts make this kind of re-feeding impractical and it might just make you feel sick. By all means experiment with peri-nutrition during strength-training sessions or yomps but, for boot runs and troop phyz workouts, peri-nutrition is more likely to cause digestive upset and curtail your exercise endeavours.

Weight Management

Being overweight can severely hamper your performance. Try doing pull-ups, burpees or running while wearing an 11.5 kg (25 lb) weighted vest to see just how much being overweight impacts on your ability to move well.

While this book is not designed to be a guide to weight loss, you will probably experience some changes in body composition as a result of your training and your new-found nutritional awareness. Armed forces recruits often lose staggering amounts of body fat despite eating as much as possible during their basic training. If you want to drop a little weight while using the exercise programme in this book, it is very important that you don't try to combine this vigorous programme with an overly restrictive diet. Remember that food is fuel and – like our previously mentioned Formula One racing car – if you don't have enough petrol in the tank, you won't even finish the race!

Diet is a dirty four-letter word! It implies a short-term fix for what is often the result of years of under-exercising and overeating. Like a get-rich-quick scheme, diets often promise much but deliver very little. All diets that promise large amounts of weight loss in a short space of time will probably have a number of factors in common:

- Very low calorie intake
- Unpleasant food choices
- Unsustainable eating regime
- Exotic food recommendations
- Unsocial eating patterns

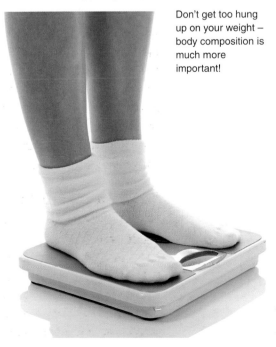

Don't get too hung up on your weight – body composition is much more important!

All in all, while virtually every diet that limits your food intake will work, it will only work for as long as you can stick with it! Once you 'fall off the wagon', as you inevitably will do after eating nothing but eggs and grapefruit or cabbage soup for a month, you will quickly revert to your old eating habits and regain all the weight you lost and a whole lot more. This is commonly referred to as yo-yo dieting and is the result of something called the starvation response. A conservative, sustainable approach to nutrition trumps a short-term diet every single time.

The Starvation Response

Once upon a time, your ancestors roamed the plain and forests, seeking food. They hunted and gathered, scrounged and foraged. When food was plentiful they got fatter and when food was scarce they got skinny. To help them live as long as possible during periods of reduced food intake, nature developed the starvation response. This response essentially ensured that, in periods of short food supply, your ancestors' metabolism slowed down and their fat stores lasted as long as possible so that they survived until their next glut of food was available. When food availability increased, their bodies were 'primed' for fat storage and any calorific excess was quickly converted to adipose tissue in case food became scarce again.

This response was essential in the past but, despite no longer having the need to hunt and gather, and an almost limitless supply of food, your body still has the same instincts and, if food supplies are drastically reduced, it still goes into starvation mode. This means that an overly aggressive reduction in food intake will result in a slowed metabolism, muscle atrophy or shrinkage, and improved fat storage ability so that, when you fall off the wagon, you actually gain back more fat than you lost. Your body has no idea that you are voluntarily reducing your food intake – it perceives the lack of food as a threat to survival and responds by ensuring that you end up fatter and better able to weather subsequent food shortages. Hardly conducive to losing a few post-Christmas or pre-summer inches!

A Modern Dilemma

Modern life is lived at a fast pace – whatever you want, you want it now! Modern diets are designed to deliver rapid results but unfortunately these types of diet do not work in synergy with your biology. It's also worth considering that most diets have a fiscal value attached to them – in other words, someone wants to make money from you! This might mean that you have to buy a book, subscribe to a magazine, buy certain food products or splash out on special dietary supplements. If you think about it logically, a diet should actually *reduce* your food bill, not *increase* it, as you should be eating less and therefore spending less!

Cashing in at the Fat Bank

Although there is more to weight loss than simple calories in versus calories out (a subject that deserves another entire book), one of the most important factors in weight management is creating an energy deficit. By going 'overdrawn' at the calorie bank, your body will be forced to dip into its fat stores to provide you with energy. If you try to make too big a fat-calorie withdrawal you'll trigger the dreaded starvation response, but a small withdrawal won't set the alarm bells ringing and should result in slow, steady, painless and sustainable fat loss. It's like a behind-the-lines commando operation – sneak in without tripping the alarm and the enemy will be none the wiser. Make too much noise and reveal your presence? Remember only to tell them your name, rank and serial number!

Creating a calorie deficit

There are three ways you can create a calorie deficit:

1. Reduce your food intake.
2. Increase your activity levels.
3. Reduce your food intake *and* increase your activity levels.

Almost every study on weight loss indicates that option 3 is the best. Relying on diet restriction alone usually leaves you hungry; exercise alone only really works on the days you actually perform your workout and, if you skip a workout, your weight loss is likely to stall. Combining a modest calorie restriction with regular physical activity won't leave you hungry and won't require you to take up full-time residence in the gym. It's a case of 1+1=3!

By simply following the exercise programmes detailed earlier in this book and eating sensibly but well, you will have no problem getting down to a healthy weight. You'll look great, feel great and be able to perform well, but if you have aspirations to get 'ripped' – a state where body fat levels are so low you look like a walking anatomy chart – you may need to make a more concerted effort with your nutritional approach.

Tweaking the programme for fat loss

So you are eating a little less and following the programme diligently, but you want to get your body fat levels low enough that you can display your hard-earned six-pack! There's nothing wrong with having some 'show' to accompany your 'go'. With a couple of very simple tweaks, you can increase your fat-burning potential and rid your body of that pesky ab-obscuring fat.

- **Reduce carbohydrate intake and increase protein intake.** Doing this will lower the amount of insulin your body produces. Insulin suppresses fat burning and promotes fat storage. You won't be eating any less – just regulating your blood glucose and therefore your insulin levels. Fill up on veggies, cut down on grains and pile on the protein. Protein also has a metabolism-boosting effect above and beyond that of carbohydrate, which can help with weight management. Consume the majority of your carbohydrate calories before and after exercise. The rest of the time, keep your carb intake low.

- **Increase your NEPA (Non-Exercise Physical Activity).** This is another way to increase your daily energy expenditure by simply being more active. It's not exercise but merely an increase in daily movement that won't impact on your exercise routine. Walk for 30 minutes after dinner, wash your car by hand, use the stairs and not the lift, do some gardening or DIY – just try to move more. The more you move, the greater your calorie withdrawal will be and the more you will dip into your fat banks!

Bodyweight versus body fat

'Weight management' and 'losing weight' are common enough terms but are actually often used incorrectly. When you hop on the scales, the readout tells you your weight in kilograms or stones and pounds, but it tells you very little about what that weight *consists of*. Your actual body composition is far more important than your scale weight. Your body is made up of a variety of substances including bone, muscle, fat, water and skin. There are also numerous chemicals stored in your body that contribute to your overall weight. You can lose weight by reducing bone mass, muscle mass, fluid levels, glycogen (carbohydrate) stores and, of course, fat. The thing is that scale weight doesn't actually reflect what you have lost. While it *might* be fat mass, you can't be sure. This is why purposeful weight loss should really be referred to as fat loss.

The term 'weight loss' is so ingrained in many people's psyche that the only aspect of their health and fitness they are interested in is their weight. Weight loss by any means is celebrated, but any kind of weight gain is vilified. Unfortunately, most diet information focuses on rapid and dramatic weight loss and seldom mentions fat loss. In the following example, you'll see typical statistics for a heavily muscled sportsman and a lightly muscled desk-jockey. According to both weight and body mass index, subject B is the healthier. However, although subject A is significantly heavier, his body fat percentage is much lower and, as a result, it is he who is likelier to be healthier.

Subject A – rugby player	Subject B – sedentary
95 kg	68 kg
Height 1.85 m	Height 1.70 m
Body Mass Index 27.77	Body Mass Index 23.53
Body fat percentage 13%	Body fat percentage 28%

Body Mass Index or BMI (weight in kilograms divided by height in metres squared) is the relationship between your height and your weight and is commonly used as an indicator of health. But BMI does not take into account *what makes up* your bodyweight, as those with higher than average amounts of muscle can seem to be overweight despite having relatively low body fat levels. In fact, lighter subject B is carrying twice the percentage of fat of subject A despite weighing considerably less and having a 'better' BMI score.

Throw away your scales and grab a tape measure!

So now you know that your scale weight isn't all that important, how can you monitor your fat loss? One option is to get your body fat levels assessed using skin fold callipers. While this method of assessment will provide an accurate picture of your body composition, it can also be very invasive and is not readily accessible. Another option is to purchase biometric scales that use electrical impedance to assess your body fat levels. The trouble with these devices is that they lack consistency and readings can vary hugely from one test to the next, depending on numerous factors including your hydration level and body temperature.

A much better and simpler option is to track loss by external measurement- so-called girth measurements. If you find you are losing centimetres/inches around your hips and/or abdomen but your bodyweight is remaining fairly static, you can be assured that you are losing fat while gaining muscle. If your waist is getting bigger it's safe to assume you are gaining fat as there are no appreciable muscles in that area that will get much bigger. While this simple method of monitoring will not reveal your body fat percentage, it will give you sufficient feedback on whether your exercise and nutrition regime is taking you towards or away from your body composition goals. If weight (sorry – fat) loss is your goal, use the chart below to track your bodyweight, waist and hip measurements.

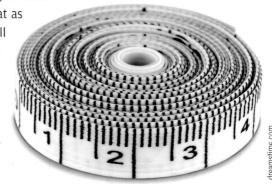

Track girth as well as weight.

Date	Hip measurement	Waist measurement	Weight

Resist the temptation to weigh and measure yourself too often. Once every 10 days to 2 weeks is plenty. Make sure you perform your testing at the same time of day and under the same conditions, i.e. using the same scales, with an empty stomach, bowel and bladder, while wearing the same clothes. Position the tape measure in exactly the same location to avoid any false readings. The actual position of the tape measure is secondary in importance to consistency, so make sure you perform your measurements in an identical fashion each and every time.

Supplements

Since time immemorial, man has been looking for ways to increase his physical prowess. Sports science might sound like a relatively new invention but the reality is that the science of ergogenics or performance enhancement is almost as old as mankind itself. Some of the earliest ergogenic aids can be traced back to early fighting forces looking for an advantage over their enemies. The gladiators of ancient Rome used herbs to reduce anxiety, increase aggressiveness and dull pain in preparation for mortal combat in the arena. Vikings ingested large amounts of alcohol and a herb called bog myrtle in the belief that it made them more aggressive and powerful. These Vikings were consequently known as Berserkers and the term 'going berserk' is derived from descriptions of their fighting prowess. The ancient warriors of Sparta are purported to have consumed dried bulls' testicles in an effort to make them stronger and more virile. Although the hormone testosterone was not identified and isolated until around 1890, the Spartans knew that castrated animals grew less massive and powerful than those left 'fully equipped', and deduced that what was good for the bull would be good for them. Whether or not ingesting dried bulls' testicles improved serum testosterone levels in Spartan warriors is unclear but, as

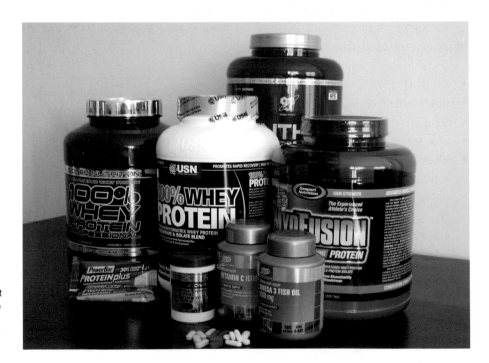

Supplements are not essential but may be useful if you are eating, sleeping and training properly.

with many forms of medication, the placebo effect can be very powerful indeed! More recently, Nazi Germany is alleged to have given anabolic steroids to frontline storm troopers to make them stronger and more resistant to fatigue and to increase aggression. One such steroid, Dianabol, has consequently been described as the 'breakfast of champions' because of its ability to increase muscle mass and strength.

For some reason, many people assume that, if you exercise, you have to take supplements. This is the fault of the glossy fitness magazines and especially those dedicated to bodybuilding. Supplementation is a purely personal choice. If you feel you need a bit of a 'leg up' then supplementation may give you the boost you need, but sports supplements cannot perform miracles and make up for a poor diet, lack of training intensity or inconstancy. If your diet is spot-on, you are training hard and regularly and getting adequate rest and recuperation, you may benefit from sports supplements. If, however, the rest of your life is a mess, not even the best, most effective supplements will make a blind bit of difference to your fitness or physique.

If you do decide to use supplements, focus your attention on ones that have been on the market for a while. If a product has been on sale for more than a few years, it means it has high enough sales to suggest that it actually works! Flash-in-the pan products that are on the shelves one week and in the bin the next have probably failed to deliver any meaningful results.

Although not exhaustive, consider this list as a good jumping-off point for supplements and please don't think I'm suggesting you have to go and buy any or all of these products. This list exists solely to steer you towards products that have stood the test of time and are more likely to actually work.

Remember, supplements are just that – supplemental to and not replacements for an already good diet.

- Creatine
- Branch chain amino acids (BCAAs)
- HMB
- Zinc and magnesium (ZMA)
- Whey protein
- Protein and energy bars
- Energy gels
- Sports drinks
- Glutamine
- L-carnitine
- Tribulus terrestris
- Multivitamins and minerals

Now you know how to fuel your workouts to eat for success, it's time to move on to how to use the strength of your mind to overcome the weaknesses of your body!

CHAPTER EIGHT

Motivation

Tips and techniques to keep you on the path

Setting exercise targets can help keep you motivated.

Exercising without a goal is a bit like going on a yomp without a map – although you are moving over the ground, you have no way of knowing if you are heading towards or away from your ultimate objective: 'I don't know where we're going, but we're making good time.' There's nothing wrong with training for training's sake *but*, in numerous psychological studies, it has been shown again and again that those exercisers who are working towards clearly defined goals are far less likely to drop out of exercise.

Recruits in training have the luxury of a Physical Training Instructor to keep them motivated. They'll be encouraged, bullied, coerced and bribed to keep going regardless of how tired they are feeling. The rest of us have to rely on our internal PTIs to ensure we don't skip workouts and exercise as effectively as possible. Some people, a very lucky few, are self-motivated and come rain, shine or snow they will find the necessary 'get up and go' to get their workouts done. For these people, the process of getting fit is often as important as actually improving their fitness levels. The rest of us … we'd rather be tucked up in bed or down the pub instead of doing yet another set of burpees in the rain!

One of the best ways to increase your self-motivation is through goal-setting. Goal-setting helps you focus your mind on the task in a hand, and strong goals can help drive you forwards when your body is yelling 'stop!' Elite athletes, high-flying business people and just about all professionals in between use goal-setting to help focus their efforts and keep them motivated. Using the yomping analogy, having clear-cut goals is like having a well-drawn map that will show you where you are currently, where you are going and how you are going to get there.

Get Smart

While arbitrary goals such as 'get fit' or 'lose weight' are better than no goals at all, goal-setting is much more effective if you can attach quantifiable values to what you are trying to achieve. Rather than saying that you 'want to get fit', decide on *how* fit you want to be, what you want to be able to achieve with your new-found fitness and when you want to achieve it by. This structured approach to target-setting is called SMART goals. SMART goals put the flesh on the bones of your otherwise vague aims. 'Lose weight' becomes 'lose X pounds in 8 weeks'. It's much easier to judge the success of your efforts when you have specific and finite targets to work towards. SMART goals roll out like this:

S – Specific. Try to set precise goals as opposed to vague concepts. Rather than decide that you want to be able to perform more press-ups or get stronger, decide *how many* press-ups you would like to be able to do, or what weights you would like to be able to lift.

M – Measurable. Make sure you can quantify your goal. Attach a figure to it to help you focus. For example, if you want to get aerobically fitter, specify a distance or time that you want to be able to run. If you can't measure it, how will you know whether you've reached your goal or not?

A – Achievable. Don't set yourself up to fail. Goals should be challenging but not beyond the realms of possibility. If you have never run a step in your life, the goal of running a 3-hour marathon in 12 weeks' time is not achievable. Be realistic; take into account where you are both physically and mentally and set goals that are just within your reach. Once you have met your first set of goals, you can select loftier ones. Every Olympic champion started off by wanting to win their school championship.

R – Recorded. Write your goals down and refer to them often. Whenever you feel as though your motivation is waning, dig out your goals and remind yourself why you are training. If it's a weight-loss goal, why not stick it to the fridge as a constant reminder of why you shouldn't scoff that big piece of cheesecake?

T – Time-bound. Set a timeframe to your goals. This may be a few short weeks or several years depending on the size of the goal you have set for yourself. If a goal is going to take you more than 3 months to achieve, set yourself intermediate goals that you can tick off as you progress towards completing your end goal. You are more likely to succeed if you break big goals down into short-, medium- and long-term 'stepping stone' goals.

Here are a couple of examples of SMART goals put into practice. There is a blank chart for you to use so you can perform the same process but, if you prefer not to write in this book, feel free to photocopy the chart or write your goals out on a piece of paper. Regardless of where you write your goals down, it is essential that you put pen to paper and get your goals 'out there'. If you want an extra dose of motivation, share your goals with the world by telling your friends and family or, alternatively, starting an online training blog. By making your goals public you are even more unlikely to backslide or quit. Peer pressure is a wonderful thing!

Example 1 – 'getting better at press-ups'

	Short	Medium	Long
S	Perform 30 press-ups in a single set	Perform 60 press-ups in a single set	Perform 100 press-ups in a single set
M	Yes – during fitness testing	Yes – during fitness testing	Yes – during fitness testing
A	Yes – by focusing on press-ups in my training 3 times a week	Yes – by focusing on press-ups in my training 3 times a week	Yes – by focusing on press-ups in my training 3 times a week
R	Yes – in my training diary and in fitness testing log sheets	Yes – in my training diary and in fitness testing log sheets	Yes – in my training diary and in fitness testing log sheets
T	One month	Three months	Six months

Example 2 – 'I want to lose weight'

	Short	Medium	Long
S	Lose 2.25 kg (5 lb) total	Lose 4.5 kg (10 lb) total	Lose 9 kg (20 lb) total
M	Yes – fortnightly weigh-ins	Yes – fortnightly weigh-ins	Yes – fortnightly weigh-ins
A	Yes – averages around ½–1 kg (1–2 lb) per week	Yes – averages around ½–1 kg (1–2 lb) per week	Yes – averages around ½–1 kg (1–2 lb) per week
R	Yes – by recording weight loss in training diary	Yes – by recording weight loss in training diary	Yes – by recording weight loss in training diary
T	One month	Two months	Four months

As you can see, the arbitrary goals of 'getting better at press-ups' and 'losing weight' have been put through the SMARTer goal-setting mill and, as a result, our new recruit will have much more focus. Every meal consumed and workout performed will be a step towards achieving something much more tangible.

What Happens When You Reach Your Goals?
First - congratulate and reward yourself! Then simply raise the bar and set yourself new challenges. You could stick with the same goal and try to challenge yourself even further, for example even more press-ups, or you could focus on a different element of your fitness, such as increasing your flexibility, or a particular race you would like to compete in.

Your personal goal-setting chart

	Short	Medium	Long
S p e c i f i c			
M e a s u r a b l e			
A c h i e v a b l e			
R e c o r d e d			
T i m e- b o u n d			

More Motivational Strategies

While goal-setting is a very powerful motivational tool, there are a few other strategies that you can employ to help keep you on the straight and narrow path to physical fitness. Each of the following strategies has been tested in the trenches of commercial gyms, where typically only 30% of new joiners are still attending regularly 3 months after signing on the dotted line. The 70% dropout is actually good news for gym owners as it means they can 'resell' unused memberships over and over again so, while they may have a total membership of several thousands, in reality, only a few hundred actually attend the gym on a regular basis. Good news for the gym owners' pockets; bad news for the nation's waistline, blood pressure and overall fitness levels!

Training and Nutrition Diaries

I've kept training diaries since I was a 16-year-old wannabe bodybuilder. I have dozens of little notebooks that I've dragged to every gym workout to record exercises, sets, reps and weights. As a triathlete, I kept training diaries detailing every metre swum and every mile cycled or run. Even now, despite no longer training for any competitive sport, I still record all my workouts in my latest training diary. Why? Because every blank page means a skipped workout and I *hate* blank pages!

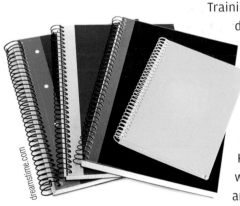

Recording your workouts has been shown to enhance motivation.

Training diaries are also essential for recording progress, spotting upward or downward trends in performance and making sure each workout is as productive as possible. Unless you have a photographic memory, how will you know how much weight you lifted or how fast you ran from one week to the next? Remember that progression is the key to increasing your fitness and strength. If you don't add a little more weight to the bar, complete an extra rep or run a little further or faster, your fitness gains will stagnate and you'll find yourself on the dreaded plateau. Keep a training diary and you'll never have to worry about remembering what weights to lift or how many reps to perform – it'll be there in black and white. Personally, I use small, hard-backed A5 notepads for my training diaries, but you should use whatever is convenient. There are some training diary sheets near the end of this book for you to photocopy and use. There is no need to become a fanatical record keeper – just make sure you make a note of the important information so you can adjust your subsequent workouts accordingly.

Nutrition diaries can be useful if you are trying to lose fat or gain muscle weight. Weight loss requires a calorie deficit while weight gain requires a calorie surplus. This means you need to know roughly what you are eating on a day-to-day basis. While I don't think you need to weigh and measure all of your food, you should have a rough idea of what you are putting into your body so that you can establish a nutritional baseline and make alterations based on your progress. If your weight isn't changing then you need to make dietary alterations.

In weight management, particularly with weight loss, there is a phenomenon called the 'mouth-mind gap'. The mouth-mind gap describes how some people forget what they have eaten and consequently overeat. The mouth-mind gap is widest when you are sitting watching TV, driving your car, or otherwise distracted and happily snacking away. Before you know it, that small handful of nuts has morphed into a whole bag but, oddly, you don't remember eating them at all! Not surprisingly, this results in weight gain rather than weight loss. Writing down everything you eat means that you cannot hide from the truth. If your weight is not changing it's because of what you are (or, in the case of purposeful weight gain, are not) eating!

I don't suggest that you keep a food diary forever, but doing so for a week every month or two helps to focus your mind on exactly what you are eating. Most people tend to eat a fairly cyclic diet so periodically tracking your nutritional intake should highlight emerging trends. There are also numerous online nutrition trackers so, if you *really* want to know what you are putting into your body, try entering a few typical days' food consumption into one of these programmes and see what's what.

Decision Balance Sheets

Life is full of choices - steak or chicken, beer or wine, ice cream or yoghurt, workout or watch TV? Each decision offers advantages and disadvantages. The trick is to choose the option that is going to take you closer to your ultimate fitness goal and not further way! Rather than just going with your gut feeling, you can use the decision balance process to make a more informed choice.

Perhaps you are thinking that you'll skip this week's yomp in favour of going to the pub instead ... weigh up the pros and cons of this decision using the decision balance sheet.

Skipping workout – Pros	Skipping workout – Cons
I will see my friends	I won't get any fitter
I can have a few beers	I will probably gain weight from the beer and the subsequent takeaway on the way home
We can watch football on the TV	I will have to try to catch up missed workout so will have less time to relax next week
	I'm going to feel guilty about missing workout
	I'll end up with a hangover and feel terrible for the next 1–2 days
	I'm going to let my training partner down
	There will be a blank page in my training diary

More often than not, it soon becomes obvious which choice is most likely to help drive you towards your goals. The thing is, you know which choice is the most sensible one, but it's only when you take a couple of minutes to write it down that you realize how the benefits and disadvantages weigh up. Think of a decision balance sheet as a way to confirm what you know is true – it's not always easy developing your fitness but, in the long run, it's worth every sacrifice. Anyway, you can always go to the pub after your workout!

Training Partners – an Army of Two

No man is an island; a problem shared is a problem halved; two heads are better than one; there is no 'I' in team … there is a long list of proverbs and sayings that suggest that going it alone is not always the best option. One of the most abiding memories I have of Marine basic training and subsequent deployments is that someone always 'had your back'. Peer encouragement was a constant and, for many recruits and soldiers, was the difference between ultimate success and failure. Knowing that you aren't suffering alone is a very powerful motivator. While you won't have a squad of like-minded individuals to train with, you can recruit a training partner to join you on your quest for fitness.

A training partner can help spot you in the gym, keep you going when you might rather stop, encourage you to perform better by cheering you on, or simply make sure you don't miss a workout because they have agreed to meet you at a specific time. The chances are very good that, on the days you are feeling sub-par and feel like taking it easy, your training partner is firing on all cylinders and will drag you kicking and screaming through a workout you might otherwise have missed. Don't worry, though: as luck would have it, you'll be in the driving seat soon enough when your training partner has an off day!

Personally I prefer training alone – I've been doing so for over 25 years and have my own workout rhythm that I like to stick to. I know when to push myself, when to back off and when I need a rest. That said, on the rare occasions I do train with someone, I usually find that I raise my game slightly, if for no other reason than because my fragile male ego forces me to! If you do decide to work out with a training partner, make sure their goals are aligned with yours and they are similarly fit. Too much of a fitness gap can mean that one of you will get to coast while the other is working their butt off! Likewise, make sure your partner's training values are similar to yours. If they are constantly late for your workouts, want to knock off early, or in any other way are unreliable, don't be afraid to train alone. You might hurt their feelings when you explain that you want to 'divorce' them as your training partner, but if your progress is being hampered by someone who is supposed to be helping you, it's the most sensible option. It's better to cut them loose than waste your valuable energy on non-productive workouts.

Cheat Days

In nutrition, cheat days are designated free days when you can relax from your strict diet and have a little of what you fancy. This isn't an excuse to try to eat your body-weight in chocolate, but merely an opportunity to indulge in a little of something that you have been denying yourself over the last week or so. Programming cheat days into your dietary plan means that, in the first instance, you have something to look forward to each week and also that nothing is completely off limits. For weight loss, occasional cheat days offer both psychological and physiological benefits and can help prevent weight-loss plateaux.

With regard to exercise, the occasional unscheduled rest day can mean that you have more energy than usual for subsequent workouts. If, for example, a workout lands on a bank holiday, why not enjoy the extra day off and then come back well rested and stronger for the next day's workout? This isn't laziness – simply a reward for your hard work to date.

If you feel like skipping a workout because you are tired you may well find that, once you get through your warm-up, you feel fine and end up having a great training session. If after warming up you *still* feel lacklustre and unenthusiastic then maybe

Training with a friend equals twice the motivation!

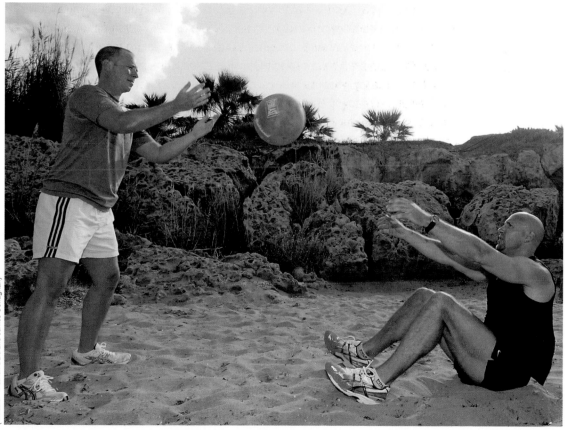

(Models – Patrick Dale and James Conaghan)

an extra day off is in order. By applying the 'warm-up test' you can see if you are just being lazy or are genuinely in need of an extra day of rest. Alternatively, if you feel you aren't firing on all cylinders, consider performing the prescribed workout at a slower pace, or complete only half the training volume. An easy day today may mean a better day tomorrow.

On the rare days I feel too tired to train at full intensity, I warm up for 10 minutes and then cool down for 10 minutes and miss out my main session entirely. This abbreviated workout infuses my brain and muscles with fresh oxygen, stretches my muscles and mobilizes my joints without taxing my recovery abilities. I usually find that the next day's workout is an absolute belter as a result!

A Word on Overtraining

There is no denying that exercise is good for you but, like so many things, too much can be harmful. How much is too much? It's very individual and depends on your tolerance to exercise, recuperative abilities, general health and nutritional status, but if you are taking too much out of your body and not putting enough back in, overtraining syndrome is likely to be the result.

Overtraining syndrome is a chronic condition that can affect anyone from Olympic athletes to recreational exercisers. Once you have developed overtraining syndrome it can be very difficult to shake off, so it is best avoided altogether. Overtraining syndrome normally presents with some or all of the following symptoms. If you are suffering from more than three of the signs listed below you may be in danger of developing overtraining syndrome and should take the appropriate action.

1. Your resting heart rate is 10% or more higher than usual.
2. Your legs feel tired, sore or heavy all of the time.
3. You are getting fatter despite training and eating properly.
4. You experience an increased incidence of minor injuries, aches and/or pains.
5. Workouts that you previously completed easily are now major challenges.
6. You experience mood swings.
7. There is a noticeable decrease in your strength and/or fitness.
8. You experience a loss of appetite.
9. Your enthusiasm for training is decreased.
10. Despite feeling tired all the time, you are unable to get a good night's sleep.
11. You are ill more often than usual.
12. You experience digestive upset more than usual.

Before you start to worry too much, chronic overtraining is the result of a very prolonged period of excessive exercise and insufficient rest. You aren't going to develop it overnight and it isn't contagious! However, if you notice a trend of poor workouts in your training diary (I told you it was important to keep one) then it may be worth taking pre-emptive action to avoid a full-on crash. Strategies for avoiding overtraining syndrome include the following:

1. Consume a good-quality post-workout meal or drink after every training session.
2. Get enough sleep.
3. Reduce your stress levels.
4. Get regular sports massages.
5. Back off your training whenever you begin to feel overly tired.
6. Consume sufficient carbohydrates to fuel your activities.
7. Consume sufficient protein for muscle repair and growth.
8. In addition to the macronutrients, consume adequate micronutrients and water to ensure your body has all the resources it needs for post-exercise adaptation, recovery and repair.
9. Listen to your body and don't be a slave to the programme – if you need more rest days or easier workouts, then take them!
10. Scale the workouts in the programme to suit your individual fitness needs.
11. Increase the duration, frequency, volume and intensity of your workouts gradually.
12. Take periodic breaks of 5–7 days from training. One week off every 12 or so will not result in lost fitness, but may actually enhance your physical performance.

CHAPTER NINE

Frequently Asked Questions

Straightforward answers to common fitness and health questions

I've tried to make this book as comprehensive as possible so that you can develop a high level of fitness for anything life throws at you. However, the world of health and fitness information is huge and getting bigger every day. With this in mind, I have provided answers to some of the most common training, health and nutrition questions that I am asked in the hope that I can address any concerns that may arise as a result of reading this book. If you have any additional questions, please email me at patrickdale.militaryfitness@hotmail.com and I will endeavour to answer them for you.

Question 1
Some exercises in your programme seem a little old-fashioned – why have you chosen these particular exercises?

I have selected each exercise on its individual merits and its accessibility. While there are hundreds of exercises to choose from, some are very hard to learn and perform correctly. For example, the power clean and the kettlebell swing target similar muscle groups but the power clean is a much more technically demanding exercise that can take a long time to learn. Wherever possible, I have selected exercises with which you will already be familiar, or can learn easily. The final common denominator for all the exercises selected is effectiveness. Each one provides maximum 'bang for your buck' and will deliver excellent results when performed with sufficient intensity.

Question 2
I don't belong to a gym. Will I still be able to follow your programme?

I *own* a gym and yet prefer to do most of my training at home! You can get a great workout using the equipment options described in Chapter 6. Use sandbags, rocks, water barrels, resistance bands or suspension training equipment for the strength workouts. Also, most of the troop phyz workouts use very little in the way of workout gear. My main aim in this book is to show you how you can develop phenomenal fitness using a very low-tech approach to training. The military have been doing this for years so there is no reason why you can't do the same!

Question 3

I have no interest in joining the armed forces and just want to get fit and lean. Is your programme still suitable for me?

Most definitely! This programme is born out of my joint areas of professional interest – fitness training and serving in the armed forces. You can take the workouts outlined in this book and develop a high degree of physical fitness and strength even if you have no intention of ever joining up.

Question 4

What should I do if I am unable to perform one or more of the exercises detailed in the workouts?

If you can't perform an exercise because of pain, I strongly suggest that you see your doctor for a proper diagnosis. If your inability is a consequence of lack of fitness or strength, simply scale the exercise down to suit your current abilities. For example, if you can't do full press-ups, bend your legs, place your knees on the floor and perform three-quarter press-ups instead. Finding burpees impossible? Eliminate the press-up and/or jump. As the weeks go by and your fitness increases, you will find you are able to perform the exercises as prescribed but, in the meantime, just work within your own personal limits.

Scale the workouts to suit your individual fitness requirements.

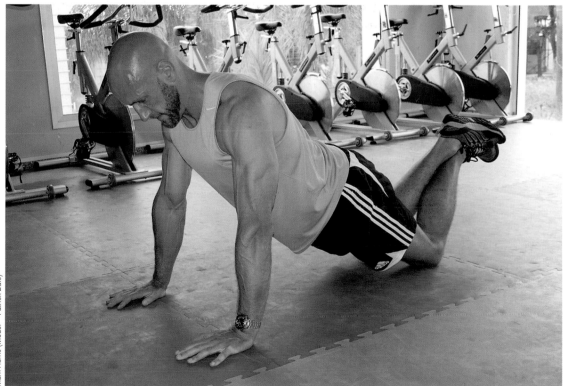

Mark Hume (Model – Patrick Dale)

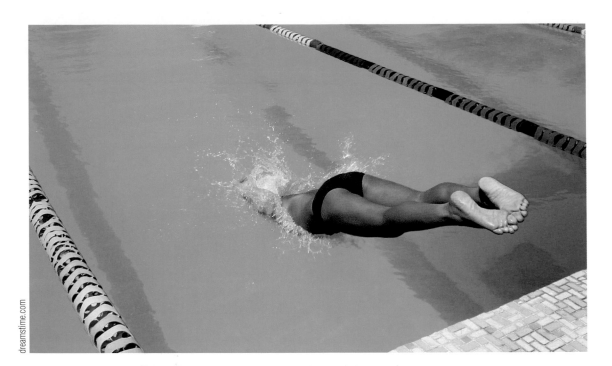

Swimming is a viable alternative to running.

Question 5

I hate running! Can you suggest a substitute for the boot run workouts?

Feel free to substitute swimming, cycling or rowing for running. Just make sure you split your total training time in half and do your very best to perform the second half of the workout as fast as you can.

Question 6

What if I can't perform the prescribed number of repetitions listed in the workouts?

You have a number of options: reduce the number of reps to a more manageable level, keep the reps the same but perform an easier version of the exercise in question, or grind out all the reps but take periodic breaks. For example, if a workout calls for you to do one set of 20 reps of press-ups, perform 10, take a breather, perform 5 and another breather and then do the final 5 to total 20. This is called a broken set. As you get fitter, reduce the number of breaks you take until you are able to complete all the prescribed reps.

Question 7

How much weight should I lift in the strength workouts?

I can't really answer this for every individual as everyone is different. Choose a weight that allows you stay within the prescribed range of reps or allows you to *just* complete the number of reps listed. For example, if the recommended rep range is 8–12 select a weight that allows you to do at least 8 but no more than 12. If you don't manage 8 then you selected too heavy a weight and if you can do more than 12 then it is too light. Don't train to complete failure. Instead, stop 1 rep short of complete exhaustion. Don't worry if you don't get your weights spot-on every time – with practice you'll be able to estimate with far more accuracy. Remember to perform all your reps with excellent technique and control and then, even if you have selected the wrong weight, your set will still be productive.

Question 8
My muscles are really sore after the first few workouts – am I doing anything wrong?

The common exercise terminology for sore muscles caused by exercise is DOMS – short for Delayed Onset Muscle Soreness. No one is exactly sure what causes DOMS. It might be that you have worked harder than usual, that there was a build-up of metabolic waste products which have not been effectively removed, or that there are micro-tears in your muscles ... all we do know is that DOMS is triggered by new or harder-than-usual exercise. It's not terminal, but it's not an indicator of a successful workout. It's just something that happens. To minimize DOMS make sure you cool down properly and don't increase your workout intensity or volume too dramatically. Vitamin C and fish oils may help with DOMS as these substances are anti-inflammatory, but DOMS usually subsides on its own after a few days.

Question 9
I haven't exercised in years – can I still do your programme?

Yes, but first go and see your doctor and get a full check-up. Then, if the doctor says it's OK to carry on, scale down the workouts according to your current fitness levels. You should see some quite dramatic improvements in your fitness levels over the next few weeks, but it is important you 'make haste slowly' in order to avoid excessive and prolonged DOMS, reduce the likelihood of injury and avoid losing motivation.

Question 10
What happens once I have completed the 12-week programme?

I suggest you repeat the programme but increase the duration of the boot runs and yomps, try to work harder during all of the troop phyz workouts and increase the weights used for the strength-training workouts. Alternatively, try to design your own 12-week plan using the other principles, exercises and methods described in the book.

Question 11

With regard to meal frequency – how often should I eat?

As with the best time to exercise, the best time to eat is when it suits you! There are advantages to eating every 3 hours but, if your boss frowns on you eating chicken legs or sipping protein shakes when you are sitting at your desk, polyphasic eating schedules are not going to work for you. Make sure you start your day with a good breakfast consisting of protein, slow-release carbohydrates and healthy fats and try to continue eating well throughout your day. If this ends up being two more biggish meals or five smaller ones, so be it. Do your best to eat frequently but if this isn't practical then do the best you can. Just about everyone can manage two good meals and two reasonable snacks per day. This may take some planning and require preparing food in advance, but your results will be all the better if you do. The bottom line is - make sure that, one way or another, you eat enough to fuel your workouts.

Question 12

What is your advice for post-exercise meals? Are drinks or real food best?

Both options can work - it's a matter of personal preference. Post-exercise shakes are quick and convenient but can also be costly. A 'real' meal is often the cheaper option but not always the most convenient. Some exercisers lose their appetite immediately after exercise, so a shake would work better for them. So long as you ingest a decent amount of protein and carbs in the hour or so after exercise, you will kick-start your recovery process and ensure that you make the most of your anabolic window.

Question 13

Do I need a multivitamin/multimineral supplement?

In a perfect world, you should be able to get all the micronutrients you need from 'real' food. Unfortunately, it is not always possible to eat exactly as you should and sometimes you may need to give nature a helping hand. By all means take a good-quality multivitamin/multimineral supplement as a nutritional safety-net, but remember that even the best pill will not contain all the nutrients you need for health and wellbeing.

Question 14

I have a minor injury from working out – what should I do?

First, don't ignore it. If not treated properly, minor niggles have a way of becoming major injuries. If you feel an injury come on, stop what you are doing and get some ice on the injured area. Continue to ice the injury for 10-15 minutes every couple of waking hours for the next few days. If you think your injury is more serious, seek medical attention. Once you are able to move around with little or no pain, reintroduce some very light exercise for that area and then, over the next 7-10 days, increase the volume and intensity of the exercise until you have returned to your previous levels. If at any time you experience any pain, back off and then rebuild your momentum while continuing with your ice treatment.

If your injury is to an upper limb, for example your shoulder, feel free to continue performing lower-body dominant exercises such as running or cycling. Likewise, if you have a lower-body injury, it's OK to hit the weights or otherwise work your upper body. Back injuries are a different matter altogether and much harder to work around. As your health should be your paramount concern, if you are in any doubt as to how to deal with an injury, you should seek medical advice.

Tight hamstrings? Stretch them as often as you can!

Question 15
My hamstrings are super-tight! What should I do?

Stretch! It has probably taken years for your hamstrings to tighten up, so it's going to require a concerted and consistent approach to stretching to fix the problem. I suggest stretching three to five times a day for 1-2 minutes per session for as long as it takes to increase your flexibility. Always stretch gently but progressively. I don't expect you to warm up before every stretching session, so make sure you ease into your stretches very slowly and carefully. Sports massage may also be of benefit.

Question 16
How much sleep do I need per night?

Sleep is when your body goes through the complex process or growth, repair and recovery. Quality sleep is essential for maximal fitness

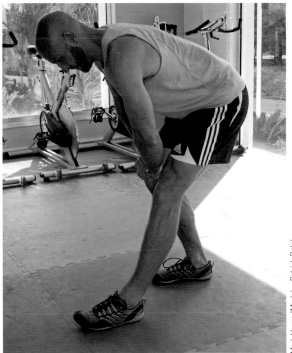

Mark Hume (Model — Patrick Dale)

gains. That being said, I averaged around 4 hours' sleep per night during my 30-week Royal Marines basic training and often had less on deployment. It's far from ideal but you can survive for a long time on relatively low amounts of sleep. Shoot for 6-8 hours per night and, if possible, enjoy a 20-30 minute 'power nap' in the middle of the day to aid your recovery from exercise.

dreamstime.com

A good night's sleep can be the difference between recovering and not recovering after a hard workout.

Question 17

Is this programme suitable for women and men?

Most definitely! The compound nature of the exercises I have selected and the high-intensity workouts will help strengthen and firm both male and female bodies. Women lack muscle-building testosterone so while men may expect to add some muscle mass as a result of this programme, this is much less likely for women. However, the emphasis is on hip, leg and lower back exercises like squats and kettlebell swings, which also target the area that, historically, most women want to work on - the butt.

Question 18

I can't commit to training five days per week but I like the look of your programme – how can I modify it to fit a four-times-a-week training schedule?

Given your limited schedule, I would cut out one of the troop phyz workouts. Perform one boot run, one strength workout, one troop phyz workout and one yomp per week. You should still make excellent fitness gains using this abbreviated version of the programme.

Question 19

Some of the exercises and workout methods you have described are not part of the 12-week programme. Can I still use them?

Most definitely! If you really like a particular exercise, for example hammer swings, feel free to incorporate it into one of the troop phyz workouts or use it as a 'finisher'

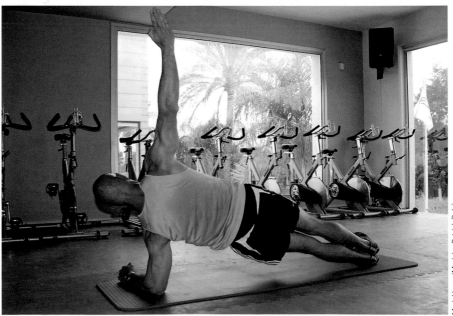

Not all the exercises in this book are featured in the workouts, so feel free to add them if you want some variation.

Mark Hume (Model – Patrick Dale)

after strength training. Try not to add too much extra work into the programmes though – if you feel you need to increase the volume of the training you are performing, I would suggest you aren't pushing yourself as hard as you should. Despite some of the workouts being very short, you should still finish each one feeling that you gave it your all.

Question 20
Will this programme help me get fit for my sport?

Whether you play rugby, soccer or basketball, or are a boxer or a runner, this programme will definitely help increase your general conditioning for your chosen sport. On the downside, the full weekly (5-day) training schedule may mean that you have limited time and recovery resources to train for your sport as well. I suggest dropping one troop phyz workout (as described in Question 18) so that you have sufficient time and energy for practising your sport. This programme is ideal as an off-season training regime for most sports but, because of the relatively high frequency and high intensity of exercise, it may be too much if you play your sport competitively every week. Adjust the programme according to the time and energy you have available, but monitor yourself for any signs of overtraining, as described in Chapter 8.

You'll be fit for any sport if you follow the 12-week programme in this book!

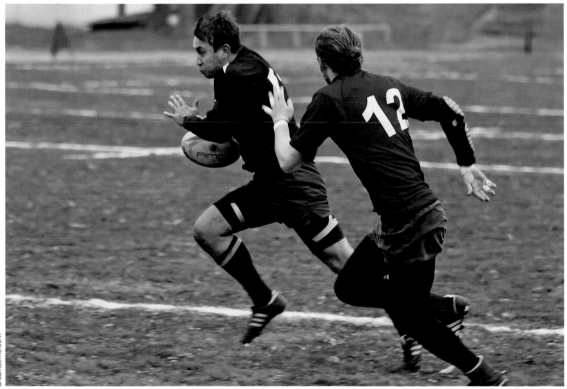

dreamstime.com

Question 21

Will this programme help me to 'bulk up'?

While this programme is not designed to be a bodybuilding plan, you may well gain an appreciable amount of muscle as a result of the high-intensity workouts and regular strength-training sessions. The muscle you gain can best be described as functional in that, although it will look impressive, it will also be usable. You'll find your new muscle mass allows you to move better, jump higher, run faster and lift heavier weights. Improved aesthetics or physical appearance is not the aim of this programme, but is a very likely and very welcome side effect!

Question 22

What do you think of diets like the Zone, the Palaeolithic Diet, Atkins diet and Slow Carb diet?

Lose your belly by following the nutritional advice and programme in this book!

Any diet that you can stick to religiously and that you enjoy is probably a good diet. Personally, I follow a modified Palaeolithic diet and eat mainly animal proteins, vegetables, fruits and nuts and mostly avoid grains and sugar. I say 'mostly' because at weekends and immediately after training I tend to eat foods that are not strictly Palaeolithic, either as occasional treats or to restock my diminished glycogen stores. One of the reasons why there are so many diets around is that, to one extent or another, they all work!

Whenever anyone asks me for nutritional advice my answer is always the same: stick to natural foods, build each meal around protein and vegetables, add a small amount of unrefined carbohydrates like wild rice or potatoes according to your activity levels and consume plenty of healthy fats in the form of olive oil, coconut oil or other cold-pressed vegetable oils. Reduce sugar and refined grains and avoid calorie-dense beverages such as sodas and creamy coffee drinks. Follow these guidelines and you won't need to worry about the latest celebrity-endorsed diet.

Question 23

I have a bit of a belly – will performing extra ab work help flatten my stomach?

Extra ab-specific training will not make the fat on your belly melt away any faster. The only way to achieve the flat stomach you want is to lose fat by creating a calorie deficit (eat a little less and exercise a little more) and to perform irregular but effective strength-training exercises to target the muscles of your midsection. Follow the programme as it is laid out – it includes plenty of targeted exercise for your midsection. Follow the advice on weight (specifically fat) loss in Chapter 7 and you'll be well on your way to developing washboard abs!

dreamstime.com

Question 24
How fast should I aim to do the boot runs?

Pacing is an important part of the boot run workouts. The idea is to run the outward leg at an easy and comfortable speed and then run back along the same route as fast as you can. In terms of intensity, you should be running at close to your anaerobic threshold. This means that, if you were to run any faster, you'd have to slow down. Anaerobic threshold (AnT for short) is your highest sustainable aerobic pace. Think of the return leg of your boot run workouts as a race against yourself and then, chances are, you'll be working at the right level of intensity.

Question 25
I notice you haven't included any direct arm work in the strength programmes. Why is this and is it OK if I add some?

Direct arm work becomes less essential when you focus your attention on compound exercises such as pull-ups and bench presses. Your arms have to work very hard in this type of exercise and so they won't need much, if any, direct exercise. In fact, your arms tend to be the 'weak links' in pulling and pushing exercises and extra work may actually be detrimental. If you really want to add some direct arm work, for example biceps curls or triceps push-downs, add a few sets at the end of the strength workouts or after one of your other training days. Don't fall into the trap of performing direct arm work too early in your workout as you'll find that tired biceps and triceps will adversely affect your performance in the more important compound exercises. Tired biceps and chin-ups are not a good combination!

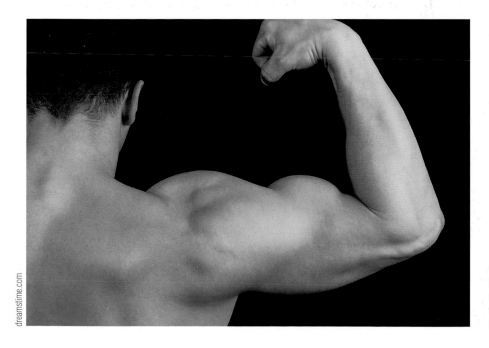

dreamstime.com

You'll build strong and functional muscle as a result of the workouts in this programme.

CHAPTER TEN

Training and Food Diaries
Charts to record your progress

You can use a notebook, Excel spreadsheet or these pages to track your exercise endeavours and food intake. Record keeping will make it much easier for you to track progress and help you stay focused. Make copies of these pages and store them in a folder or use them as templates for your notebook or spreadsheet. Whatever method of record keeping you choose, the most important thing is that you refer back to your previous notes so you can keep an eye on your progress. As we say in the forces, 'failing to plan means planning to fail', so put pen to paper or finger to keyboard and start recording your progress!

Using the Training Diary Sheets
You can use these sheets to record information about all of the workouts contained within this programme.

Workout – note the name or number of the troop phyz workout, or state whether you performed a boot run, yomp, strength-training workout or other form of training.

Exercises – if you are changing any element of the workout from the exercises listed within the programme, make a note here.

Sets/Reps – record the number of reps and sets you perform. Use shorthand if you like. For example, rather than write that you performed 5 sets of 12 reps, use the notation 5 x 12.

Weight – record the weights you used so that you can keep track of progress. Use kilograms or pounds according to your personal preference. Tracking your weights means you'll be able to see your progress and you'll know what weights to use the next time you perform this particular workout. Not all workouts use weights, so leave this box blank as necessary.

Duration – some of the troop phyz workouts are against the clock so record the time it takes you to complete them here. You can also use this box to note the duration of your boot runs and yomps. Remember that, for the boot runs, you need to record your outward time and your return time separately and your return time should generally be significantly faster!

Recovery – make a note of how long you rest between sets of strength-training exer-

	Workout	Exercises	Sets/reps	Weight	Duration	Recovery	Observations
Monday							
Tuesday							
Wednesday							
Thursday							
Friday							
Saturday							
Sunday							

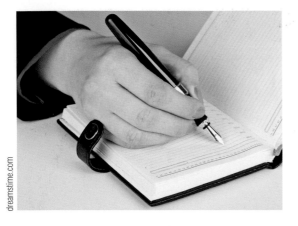
dreamstime.com

cises or laps of circuits. Try to reduce the length of your recoveries as you get fitter.

Observations - record your general thoughts about how the workout went in this box. You might include information on the weather if you feel it contributed to your performance, or make a note to remind yourself to use a heavier weight for next week's bench press workout. If you had a less-than-optimal workout because you made a mistake timing your pre-exercise meal, make a note of it so you have no excuse for making the same error again.

Record your workout performance so you can monitor your progress.

Using the Food Diary Sheets

There is no need to weigh and measure your food. Simply list the basic contents of each meal and approximate portion sizes. The aim of this exercise is not to record your calorific intake but to examine the types of food you are eating. In reality, if you eat the right *types* of food, the quantities become almost an irrelevance. Make a note of what you eat as your pre- and post-exercise meals and also make use of the mood and energy indicators.

Assess your energy and mood levels 1 hour after each meal by ticking the relevant symbol. If you are somewhere in between the specified levels, simply highlight the two symbols that best describe how you feel. For example, if, after breakfast, you feel fairly energetic and in a good mood mark both ☺ and ☺. If you are feeling slightly below average but not rock-bottom, highlight ☺ and ☹.

☺ = Feeling very happy and/or energetic
☺ = Average feelings of happiness and/or energy
☹ = Feeling unhappy and/or lacking energy

If you are getting more ☹s and ☺s than ☺s then you may need to examine your diet and act accordingly. Midday and post-eating slumps in energy and mood suggest low blood glucose levels. Low blood glucose levels can be the result of too little carbohydrate or a dip caused by the rebound effect of eating too much sugar. As a rule, stable blood glucose levels should score ☺ after ☺ after ☺!

	Meal one	Meal two	Meal three	Meal four	Meal five	Meal six
Monday						
Energy/mood	☺ 😐 ☹	☺ 😐 ☹	☺ 😐 ☹	☺ 😐 ☹	☺ 😐 ☹	☺ 😐 ☹
Tuesday						
Energy/mood	☺ 😐 ☹	☺ 😐 ☹	☺ 😐 ☹	☺ 😐 ☹	☺ 😐 ☹	☺ 😐 ☹
Wednesday						
Energy/mood	☺ 😐 ☹	☺ 😐 ☹	☺ 😐 ☹	☺ 😐 ☹	☺ 😐 ☹	☺ 😐 ☹
Thursday						
Energy/mood	☺ 😐 ☹	☺ 😐 ☹	☺ 😐 ☹	☺ 😐 ☹	☺ 😐 ☹	☺ 😐 ☹
Friday						
Energy/mood	☺ 😐 ☹	☺ 😐 ☹	☺ 😐 ☹	☺ 😐 ☹	☺ 😐 ☹	☺ 😐 ☹
Saturday						
Energy/mood	☺ 😐 ☹	☺ 😐 ☹	☺ 😐 ☹	☺ 😐 ☹	☺ 😐 ☹	☺ 😐 ☹
Sunday						
Energy/mood	☺ 😐 ☹	☺ 😐 ☹	☺ 😐 ☹	☺ 😐 ☹	☺ 😐 ☹	☺ 😐 ☹

Index